All Natural Mom's Guide to the Feingold Diet

A Natural Approach to ADHD and Other Related Disorders

By Sheri Davis

D1469000

ISBN: 978-0986254802

Scripture quotations are from the Holy Bible, New International Version (NIV) copyright @ 1978 by New York International Bible Society. Published by permission.

Edited by Cody Davis

Photographs by Annie Giambri of Maple Valley Photography

Portions of the proceeds of this book will go to Children With Hope and Destiny (CHAD), a non-profit Christian organization that helps orphaned children in Malawi, Africa. www.chad.org.mw

For more information about the Feingold Diet visit www.feingold.org or www.allnaturalmomof4.com.

On Facebook at www.facebook.com/allnaturalmom.

Or on Pinterest at www.pinterest.com/allnaturalmom4.

Acknowledgments

I would like to thank all the moms who have taught me so much over the years. Moms who have selflessly shared all they had learned over the years. Moms who had already helped their own children but chose to stick around to help other families. I often wondered why they would give of their time so graciously but soon realized we all had one thing in common: We wanted to help our kids.

It is with much gratitude that I say, "Thank you!" I am honored to have the opportunity to help other moms in the same way. Moms can change the world!

Thank you to all the other people who have sent me e-mails. You are such an encouragement to me. I never thought my blog would reach many people outside my circle of family and friends when I began. I am thankful that God did not allow our struggles to be wasted but that He uses it every day to help other families.

Thank you to Kristi Nelson and Helen Wachowiak, for being my listening ears and proofreaders to get me off and running with this book. Thank you to my prayer team for lifting this book up in prayer, praying that above all, God would be glorified.

Thank you to Cheryl Moeller for teaching me how to write a book, and that I *can* write a book. I would not be publishing a book without your awesome workshop, advice, encouragement, prayer, and support. You have a big heart! Thank you!

Last but not least, I want to say thank you to my son, Cody. Thank you for allowing me to share your story. Your story has helped many families, and I believe it will continue to do so. I love watching God form you into the young man that He is creating you to be. I am so thankful for how God is using your story to change other families' lives for the better. Without you, we'd still be eating McDonald's and Spaghettio's every day. I owe my health to you!

Thank you for your help with this book. I am so proud to be your mom, and I will always love you no matter what you do - even if you eat red dyes!

And of course, thank you to my God and King for answers to prayers, for showing us the way when we were desperate and lost, and for allowing us to be a part of your bigger story.

Soli Deo Gloria.

*Dedicated to my amazing, awesome, brilliant son Cody.
Without you, this book would not exist.*

Table of Contents

Introduction

Our family started the Feingold Diet in February, 2005 for my four-year-old son who showed major signs of ADHD. We saw amazing results within two days of following the diet. My son was a completely different child. It was like night and day. I immediately wanted to share this information with the world. I was so thankful to have stumbled upon Feingold, and thought, "This shouldn't be! This information should be readily available to every parent! Why wasn't it?"

I told everyone who would listen about the diet. Sadly, not everyone wanted to hear it, but there were parents who did. Those were the parents who were dealing with a child with ADHD and did not want to medicate.

In 2009, I started a blog, www.allnaturalmomof4.com. I wanted a place where I could share what I had learned and offer some hope and encouragement to other parents. I wrote about topics such as the GFCF (gluten and casein/dairy free) diet. I wrote about autism, supplements, food allergies, and other diets. However, I got e-mail after e-mail from desperate parents wanting to know more about the Feingold Diet.

So, in 2012 I went back to my first love (Feingold!) and decided to focus more on the Feingold Diet to help families who wanted to learn how to treat ADHD naturally--thus the reason for this book. My web site and Facebook page have many posts about the Feingold Diet. Feel free to read about the diet there. However, I wanted to put something together that was more organized and all-encompassing. I also wanted something that could be easily shared with friends and family.

This book is for those of you who would love to do the Feingold Diet, but just can't afford the membership (or can't talk your spouse into it). It is for those who want to learn more before spending the money for the program. Or maybe you do not have a child with any kind of issues, but you want to make better and more informed choices for your family. And then there will be some who are reading this out of pure curiosity and that's OK too!

The purpose of this book is not to make parents feel guilty about what they are feeding their kids. I want to inform above all else. I hope this book helps you answer the questions, "Do I want to start the Feingold Diet for my family?" or "Do I want to make some different choices in the foods that I buy?"

I believe if parents knew both what was in the foods they were feeding their kids, and how to avoid those ingredients (what foods to sub), they would make different choices at the grocery store. For example, if a parent was given two boxes of cereal to choose from – cereal A and cereal B, which would they choose? The two cereals are very similar. They have similar ingredients and taste about the same. Cereal A is preserved with a harmful chemical called BHT which is a known carcinogen and toxic to the liver and kidneys. [1] Cereal B does not contain any preservatives. Which cereal would most parents choose? It's pretty simple. Most parents would choose the cereal without the preservatives.

But most parents don't know that cereal A contains BHT because it's not listed on the ingredients. Or they don't even know what BHT is and that it is harmful. So what do you do? Keep reading!

I want to raise more awareness about the many behavioral issues caused by artificial colors, flavors, and preservatives. I want the concepts of the Feingold Diet to be on every commercial on children's television programs. I want every parent to know exactly what is in the foods they are feeding their children. I want food companies to stop marketing these harmful foods to our children. I want schools to ban additives from school lunches and class parties. I want the FDA (Food and Drug Administration) to step up and ban dyes and other dangerous chemicals from our children's foods as some other countries have already done. [2]

I want to share what I have learned - often the hard way. It's not easy raising a child with ADHD or other behavioral issues. It takes a toll on the entire family. It's definitely not easy for your child either. No child wants to misbehave, get into trouble at home or school, or get bad grades. Eating a diet free of harmful chemicals is healthier for everyone, not just kids with ADHD. I believe the Feingold Diet can radically change the dynamics of your family for the better.

Lastly, the Feingold Diet is not about eating completely natural in the sense that the food is in the original form that God created it. It's not the finest diet, it's the Feingold Diet. Feingold members use the term "natural" loosely to define a food that originated from a whole food source. Feingold does not cut out processed foods. They do not endorse eating all processed foods either though. All things in moderation. You are avoiding foods that contain specific ingredients that were made in a laboratory, have been found to cause adverse effects, especially for ADHD sufferers, and which are not found in nature.

If you're a parent in America, you know that many of the foods our kids eat are processed. The Feingold program tells you which processed foods are without some of the most harmful additives and they explain how even some truly natural foods like apples and strawberries can cause ADHD-like symptoms. Feingold also helps you avoid harmful chemicals in non-food items such as laundry detergent, soaps, and personal care products that can pose a problem for many people.

Dr. Ben Feingold, the founder of the Feingold Diet, did research that showed that people who avoided these particularly offensive additives (dyes, artificial flavors, and preservatives) and also avoided salicylates (explained in chapter five), often found their unwanted symptoms disappeared. Dr. Feingold found the diet to be particularly helpful for kids with ADHD-like symptoms.[3]

Food can cause problems and food can cure problems. If you truly want to restore health, you also need to add in those foods that can heal the body like vegetables and other plant-based foods. I do not go in to that in this book. This book is about helping families take those first baby steps to better eating. Everyone has to start somewhere. Feingold is a great first step because the program offers guidance in helping you choose foods that are free of some of the most detrimental additives, while helping your kids not feel deprived of their favorite foods by presenting artificial-free alternatives.

And for the record, I'm not a doctor, nutritionist, professional writer, researcher, scientist, or expert. I'm a mom who has over nine years of experience with the Feingold Diet. I am simply sharing what I have learned. Talk with your doctor first if you have a child on medication before taking them off or starting a new diet. I am not giving medical, financial, or legal advice. Please continue to do your own research and decide what is best for your family.

The Feingold Diet was an answer to prayer for us. I hope the concepts of the Feingold Diet will benefit your family as much as it has benefited ours.

Chapter 1

Help! Why We Started the Feingold Diet

A Star Is Born

After 22 hours of labor and four hours of pushing, my first child was born at home. He came out wide-eyed and alert, looking for his first meal. Little did I know then that food would have a monumental effect on his behavior.

He was a happy little guy, the joy of my life. However, something told me he was going to be a handful. As soon as he started walking, he started running...and never stopped. He ran everywhere, literally. He was impulsive. He had no fear. He was "all boy." He was naturally athletic and full of energy. We nicknamed him "The Energizer Bunny", as did complete strangers. He just kept going and going. He could also throw a tantrum that would put most two-year-olds to shame.

Putting him down for a nap or for the night was incredibly hard. It was the part of the day I dreaded most. He loved to eat Mickey cereal before bed (lots of dyes). It's no wonder he had trouble getting to sleep! He would stay up very late and it was difficult to get him to settle down. He would literally be jumping up and down on his bed, laughing hysterically until he would finally just collapse and go right to sleep.

To describe him as hyper was an understatement. Every time I went to the store someone would make a comment like, "Wow, I wish I had that much energy!" or "You have your hands full!" I read that kids with ADHD are often very cute with big innocent eyes that say "What me? What did I do?" That was my son. It was hard to stay mad at him for long because he was so darn cute. I think God made these kids so cute because if he didn't, millions of kids would be left on strangers' doorsteps. (OK, not really.)

This was my first child, so I figured that was just how boys were. I was determined that my next child was going to be a girl. I painted our spare bedroom pink in wishful thinking. I thought if this is how boys are, I don't want any more boys! I even read a book that detailed how to conceive the gender of your choice. (It worked!)

Off to Preschool

When my son was three, I enrolled him in preschool, mainly because I needed a break. He was very smart so I expected him to do well. It's amazing how your children's issues are suddenly magnified tenfold as soon as they start school. He was just as wild at school as he was at home.

For some reason I thought he was only acting that way for me. Maybe I was too lenient with him, or didn't discipline him enough. I thought for sure he would listen to his teachers and behave in school. After all, he wasn't a bad kid.

One day, his teacher asked to talk to me after school. I didn't stay long enough to hear what she had to say because my son had run out the door, smacking other kids' backpacks on the way out, like he often did. She made sure to call me later though. She explained that he had dumped sand on a little girl's head at recess and refused to go to time out. She said he often would not listen to the teachers. He had a hard time sitting in circle time. He was always touching the kids next to him and not paying attention. She suggested giving him consequences for his actions. Ha! - as if I never gave him consequences.

My parents told me I needed to spank him and discipline him more. They gave me a popular Christian book on disciplining kids. I read it and was even more depressed than I was before. I tried everything the book said and nothing worked. I shoved it under my bed.

I would spank him, and he'd laugh, and turn around and say "Spank me again!" or "That felt good!" I figured that wasn't going to work. It only made me feel worse. Time outs, when I could get him to stay in one spot, didn't work either. I read other books, and nothing I tried made any difference in his behavior. I figured there wasn't a book out there that had my kid figured out.

Every day on the way to school, I would say, "You're going to listen to your teachers today, right?" "You're going to be nice to the other kids, right?" I thought if I reminded him, he might actually behave. He always answered with the same reply, "I'll try." I had butterflies in my stomach every day when I went to pick him up, wondering what he might have done that day.

Trying to Cope

I was afraid his school was going to ask me to take him out of class. I couldn't handle the daily stress. I pulled him out after the first semester. I told myself that kids his age didn't need to be in school. Maybe he just wasn't ready for school, and what did he need preschool for anyway? He was already academically ahead of all his peers. Did he need socialization? This kid was a social butterfly. Shyness was not on his radar. I did feel there was some validity to my thinking, but my real reason for keeping him out of school in reality, was because of his inability to behave and control himself.

I avoided going out and play dates just weren't happening. I knew he'd have a hard time controlling himself and honestly, no one was asking. It's not that he was malicious in nature. He just had a tendency to play too rough and too wild, and sometimes ended up hurting other kids if I wasn't watching him closely.

The terrible two'-s turned in to the horrible three'-s, and by four there was no slowing down. He was still out of control. I tried to focus on his positive qualities. He had a lot. He was extremely talkative and I imagined him being a pastor and winning people to Christ. I thought about taking him to a nursing home and letting him get all of his talking out with the elderly. They'd love him. He was quite entertaining. Who was I to quench his free spirit?

The following fall, we had some missionary friends from Africa come and stay with us. I was embarrassed at how out of control he was, and how little I could do to stop him. I knew they must have been praying for him after they left. Who wouldn't?

Frustration Sets In

After another crazy Christmas party with relatives (with lots of candy dishes laying out everywhere), and the doom of school approaching, I decided it was time to do something - but what? I tolerated his behavior at home because I was used to it. Being my first child, I didn't have much to compare it with. I just figured this was how boys were. I tried to handle it as best I could but I was exhausted, frustrated, and felt like a terrible parent.

By this time, I also had another baby to take care of – a baby girl who was a complete angel. She was the complete opposite of her brother. She was quiet, content, and laid back. I didn't even need to entertain her because watching the constant activity of her brother was entertainment enough. As she got a little older, it became more apparent how different she was from my son. I started to question whether my son's behavior was normal for a child, boy or not.

I didn't want him to get into trouble at school. I knew I could not keep him out of school forever. I put him back into a different preschool. I figured I needed to face the inevitable and get him prepared for kindergarten. Maybe this time it would be different. After all, he was older now, and maybe it was just the teacher.

He was placed in a class with all boys - seven of them. I thought, great, a smaller class is just what he needs. Maybe the class from the previous year was just too big and overwhelming for him. However, he had the same behavior problems as the year before.

Searching for Answers

I started praying fervently for an answer to why he was so hyper. Why couldn't he behave? I knew his behavior was not God-honoring. If he got extended time on this earth for obeying his parents, his life was going to be very short-lived.

One day I was reading a post online from a woman who was from Africa. She said her family moved to America and she noticed a change in her boys when they started eating the typical American foods. In

Africa, her boys had no behavioral issues. All of a sudden they were extremely hyper. She said she had linked it to the red dyes in the American foods they were eating.

I did more research and discovered the Feingold Diet. I stopped when I read that the program cost $75 (at the time). I thought, "Why would I pay them when I could just do it myself?" I felt like they just wanted my money. I knew how to read. I could avoid red dyes. (I later realized how little I knew and how wrong I was!) I was too cheap to pay for the membership even though I could afford it, and I was too prideful. So, I put the Feingold Diet out of my mind.

The red dyes and the possible link to hyperactivity got me thinking though. I wasn't even sure what red dyes were. I looked on some of our foods and drinks, and there it was. He was sensitive to dairy so he was drinking pink grapefruit juice every day which contained red dye. I removed the juice and noticed he was a little calmer. My babysitter noticed too. I tried to "limit" his consumption of red dyes.

I had already noticed that every time he had candy or ice cream, he was terrible. I had tried to cut those out too. When he did have candy, I tried to give him chocolate instead, thinking that would be better than the dyes. However, he was still having problems. I asked my midwife what would cause him to be so hyper and she said, "Sugar."

I took him to a holistic doctor and she told me his problem was yeast (this was true). She also told me that he had a hypersensitivity to light and a zinc deficiency. She then told me to feed him less processed food. OK, could you be a little more specific? I left feeling I had little direction on where to go from there. How exactly do I feed him less processed food? What was I supposed to feed him?

His new preschool teacher started noticing the same behaviors we had seen at the other school. In a parent-teacher conference, she told me she saw red flags for ADHD and wrote that on his report card. She said he couldn't sit still. He had trouble concentrating and listening to instructions. His report card was awful under the behavior section, yet under the academic section, he had all high marks. I knew he was intelligent. Why couldn't he control himself?

I started thinking back to the African woman's post about red dyes. I remembered the changes I noticed when I did remove the red dye laden juice. One day, I decided to look up the words "red dye and hyperactivity" on the Internet. I came across the Feingold Diet again.

At this point, I needed help and was willing to do whatever it took to help my son. At the end of January, I signed up and ordered my Feingold membership materials which included a detailed food shopping guide, a fast food restaurant guide, and a ton of reading materials.

I was very impatient. I had to wait about two weeks to get my materials (now you can order a PDF version for quicker access). After reading some information on the Feingold web site, I knew that what I was feeding my child was causing him to be hyper and have difficulties in school, and that it was unhealthy for him. I didn't want to feed him this stuff one more day. I couldn't wait to get started!

Chapter 2

What is the Feingold Diet?

Before I go on with our story, I wanted to stop and explain fully what the Feingold Diet is all about. The Feingold Diet is best known as an ADHD diet. However, it has also been shown to help a variety of other issues as well including autism, learning disabilities, sleep disorders, allergies, asthma, Tourette Syndrome, hives, eczema, bed wetting, and more.[1] On this diet, we eliminate all artificial colors (dyes) like red #40, yellow #5, and blue #1 to name a few.

Feingold also eliminates artificial flavors and certain preservatives such as BHT (Butylated Hydroxytoluene), TBHQ (Tertiary Butylhydroquinone), and BHA (Butylated Hydroxyanisole). Feingold also addresses the issue of salicylates in stage one of the diet. Salicylates are the natural chemicals that plants produce to ward off bugs and diseases. They are found in many fruits and other foods and can cause many adverse reactions.[2]

With the Feingold Diet, you begin at stage one. During this time, you will stay away from all high salicylate foods. After seeing at least six to eight weeks of positive results (some members call this reaching "baseline"), you can add in one new stage two food at a time to see if your child reacts (more on this in chapter five).

The Feingold Association has compiled a 400-page food list (specific to several different regions of the country) that details which foods are free of these harmful chemicals. They contact manufacturers to find out exactly what is in the foods that we eat, and also list out which foods are stage one and stage two. They are constantly updating the shopping guide as new foods come on the scene and as food ingredients change. To receive the shopping guide and all the information on how to follow the diet properly, there is a yearly membership fee (more on this in later chapters).

Many Feingold members also choose to eliminate corn syrup, as they have noticed it causes behavioral issues in their kids. Corn syrup is not considered an "unaccepted" ingredient on the Feingold Diet, but the organization does specify which foods in their shopping guide contain corn syrup so it is easy to avoid. They also specify which foods contain MSG, nitrates, and a few other things that some people may react to or choose to avoid for health reasons.

The Feingold Diet opened my eyes to the fact that food has a tremendous impact on our behavior and health. Since becoming established on the Feingold Diet, we have done many diets for many reasons: food allergies, autism, seizures, Tourette Syndrome, yeast overgrowth, meltdowns, and digestive problems.

Currently, the main diets we follow are Feingold, GFCF, and the low oxalate diet, which is similar to a Feingold stage one diet. We also avoid a few other foods because of allergies or for health reasons. I have researched and contemplated many more diets. I have looked into the SCD (Specific Carb Diet), the GAPS (Gut and Psychology Syndrome) diet, a raw foods diet (Dr. Bernard Jensen), the yeast free diet (Dr. William Crook), the Body Ecology Diet (fermented foods), a digestive enzymes approach to diet, The Maker's Diet (eating according to Biblical guidelines), the blood type diet (eating according to your blood type), the liver cleansing and gallbladder diet (for me), a plant based diet (based on *The China Study*), a nutritarian diet (Dr. Joel Fuhrman), and more.

Each diet promises to cure you of something or to provide optimum health if you follow it. I have learned that there is no one diet that is the cure for everyone. Each person is different and there may be one diet that works well for one person, and another that works well for another person. This is likely because many of the diets address and fix one main problem.

Feingold is best known for addressing the issues of hyperactivity and the inability to concentrate, but it does not address the problem of yeast overgrowth. GFCF is best known as a diet for autism. [3] However, you could be following the GFCF diet correctly and still be eating dyes. I have learned to glean and implement parts of the above diets into our family's diet, but the one factor that is constant among any diet that is meant to restore health and eliminate unwanted behaviors and symptoms is the avoidance of the harmful additives that are eliminated on the Feingold Diet.

Sometimes people ask me which diet they should do for their child, GFCF or Feingold. I believe a diet free of dyes, artificial flavors, and certain preservatives (which is Feingold stage two) should be the foundation of any other diet. If you do not remove these toxins, you are skipping a very important step in the process of healing and health.

Do you have to purchase the Feingold program and follow it 100 percent? Not everyone needs to, but I will discuss that more in later chapters. However, I do believe that everyone can make better choices if they are informed.

I don't believe we were created to eat chemicals. Our bodies don't know what to do with these chemicals because they are not food. These chemicals throw our bodies into confusion. The liver has to work overtime eliminating toxic chemicals when it should be working on eliminating environmental toxins, viruses, bacteria, and precancerous cells. [4]

I believe it shows honor to God to eat foods that God provided for us, not man-made imitations. Eating a clean diet is not always easy to do logistically. At times we are stuck out on the road and we need to eat or we are invited to someone's house for dinner. God is not calling us to perfection in our food choices, but I think he does call us to make wise decisions with what we put into our bodies on a regular basis. The fact that my kids react negatively to these harmful chemicals makes that decision that much easier.

When we are informed and can make better decisions, we should. For our family, that means the food we buy and keep in our house is free of artificial ingredients. It means we make the best choices possible when eating out and socializing. We educate ourselves on what is healthy for our bodies and we act upon that knowledge. It means we choose to cook and eat at home for the majority of our meals.

We're not perfect but we try to do our best to honor God with our food choices. Dyes, artificial flavors and preservatives are a non-negotiable and my kids know it. We may occasionally eat corn syrup or MSG but it's not an every-day choice.

The Feingold Diet helps you identify which foods contain natural ingredients, derived from real food instead of chemicals originating in a lab. There are many processed foods that were made from whole foods, but you can't always tell by reading a label. Feingold helps you navigate through that maze of uncertainty and know for sure which foods are safe and acceptable for your family. If you don't purchase a Feingold membership, you can still make changes for the better. Keep reading and I'll explain how.

What's So Bad About Dyes, Artificial Flavors, and Preservatives?

Lots! My son recently did a science project on the effects of food dyes on plants. He learned a lot about the dangers of dyes, as outlined in the information below.

In an article entitled "Food Dyes: A Rainbow of Risks", The Center for Science in the Public Interest states "In addition to considerations of organ damage, cancer, birth defects, and allergic reactions, mixtures of dyes (and Yellow 5 tested alone) cause hyperactivity and other behavioral problems in some children. Because of that concern, the British government advised companies to stop using most food dyes by the end of 2009, and the European Union is requiring a warning notice on most dye-containing foods after July20, 2010." [5]

Studies on rats and mice have been done on each dye individually, but what about the mixture of several dyes? Ever read the ingredients on a bag of Skittles or Lucky Charms? Blue, red, yellow dyes all mixed together in one product.

The CSPI study also showed that no long term studies have been done on the effects of ingesting dyes. Most of the studies recorded reactions over a two year period, and some dyes were tested for even shorter periods. We know now that smoking causes cancer, but if they did tests on the dangers of smoking over only a two year period, would they show any cases of cancer? Probably not. It takes years for cancer to develop.

Most people did not start eating larger amounts of dyes until recent decades. Fifty years ago, many families cooked mostly from scratch, eating whole foods, not processed foods bought at a supermarket. Kids were not eating dyes every day like many do now. The study also did not include an in utero phase, which means we don't know the effect dyes have on a developing fetus.

The FDA has limits on the amount of carcinogens allowed to be used in one individual dye. [5] Those limits ensure that the carcinogens in the dyes will not pose a lifetime of risk greater than one cancer per one million people. However, there are no guidelines on the total amount of these products to consume each day. What amount of dyes can be "safely" ingested each day? What if your child is eating multiple dye-laden products each day and what if they do that for years? Is there a cumulative effect of eating all these dyes together over long periods of time?

Also worth noting is that the FDA's limits were set based on 1990's dye usage data, when dye usage was 50 percent lower than it is today. The limits were also set based on an adult's bodyweight, not a child's. [5]

Let's take a look at a typical child's day. For breakfast, they may have a strawberry yogurt which has been artificially colored with red dye (this may or may not be listed on the ingredients because their supplier of strawberries may add it). They brush their teeth with brightly colored toothpaste. They go to school and get hot lunch where they have red-dye laden fruit punch. After school they snack on some cheese puffs which contain yellow and red dye. For dinner, it's macaroni and cheese containing yellow dye. After dinner, the child goes to soccer practice and grabs their favorite brightly colored sports drink which contains blue dye. By the end of the day the child has consumed a rainbow of colors.

The warning labels on dyes in the United Kingdom say, "May have an adverse effect on activity and attention in children." [6] A parent reading this warning on a label is likely going to put that food back on the shelf. Instead of warning (and scaring off) consumers, big food companies like Mars and McDonald's have chosen instead to use natural colorings in countries where the warning labels are now required (not in the U.S.).

In Europe, Skittles, Starburst, and M&M's are all colored from natural sources such as red cabbage or carrot juice instead of dyes. A strawberry sundae from a McDonald's in the U.K. is colored red with strawberries instead of red dyes. [7] My son wants to go to Europe just so he can have a strawberry sundae and Skittles without dyes! You can't even order them to be shipped to the United States. If we ever go to Europe, we plan to fill our suitcases with lots of dye free candy!

In 2011, the Feingold Association and a few other agencies tried to convince the United States government to at least put warning labels on dyes. [8] It failed to pass by a couple of votes. I guess we're getting there. Hopefully we'll catch up to other countries one day and ban them altogether.

Certain dyes have already been banned in the United States. [9] I remember when they stopped making red M&M's when I was little. Even when they reintroduced red M&M's again, my friends and I would say, "Don't eat the red ones! They cause cancer!"

In a June, 2010 article entitled "CSPI Says Dyes Pose Rainbow of Risks", The Center for Science in the Public Interest states, "The three most widely used dyes, Red 40, Yellow 5, and Yellow 6, are contaminated with known carcinogens, says CSPI. Another dye, Red 3, has been acknowledged for years by the Food and Drug Administration to be a carcinogen, yet is still in the food supply." [10]

In March, 2011, Melanie Warner reported on the FDA hearings related to food dyes for CBS News. In the article, "FDA Hears From Critics on Artificial Food Dyes. Next Step: Ignore Them," Warner reports, "There's no good reason not to ban Red 3, something then-acting FDA commissioner Mark Novitch tried to do in 1984, saying the dye 'has clearly been shown to induce cancer' and was 'of greatest public health concern.' … Other dyes, namely Blue 1, Red 40, Yellow 5, and Yellow 6, are known to cause allergic reactions in some people and have shown signs of causing cancer in lab animals." [11]

And just what are dyes made of? "Artificial food dyes are made from petroleum and approved for use by the FDA to enhance the color of processed foods." [12] That's right, petroleum! It's that stuff that sometimes gets spilled in oceans and kills the ocean life. It is a crude oil product that is used in our gasoline, diesel fuel, asphalt, and tar. Mmm, give me some of that.

Some people don't want to know the ill-effects of dyes because they want to keep enjoying their favorite foods. I can understand that and that's why I like Feingold. There is often a natural substitute for a favorite food and if there isn't, you can always make it. I don't feel deprived at all by eating a diet free of these chemicals; I feel empowered.

We also need to teach all of this to our kids. Let kids learn in school what's actually in those "fruit" snacks they are eating. When people (including kids) are informed, they are more likely to make better choices. When my son was little, he would tell his friends as they were eating brightly colored candy, "That causes cancer, you know." Of course this was not the best way to convey this information. One girl was very offended and said her mother would never feed her something that would give her cancer. Well, the fact is dyes do contain carcinogenic (cancer causing) ingredients. Most people just don't know this.

In addition to being linked to cancer, dyes can also cause hyperactivity and behavior issues in many children. [12] The dyes and hyperactivity link is more commonly known information thanks to recent media coverage.

In 2008, Chicago CBS News came out to our house and aired a three-minute segment entitled, *"Food Additives Could Be Making Your Kids Hyper."* A new British study had just been published linking food dyes to hyperactivity. Below is the article that CBS News had posted on their web site. [13]

> *"Food Additives Could Be Making Your Kids Hyper"*
>
> *Cody Davis's behavior improved dramatically after his mother began restricting the food additives he eats.*
>
> *There's something in our food that could be affecting your child's behavior, and could even be causing behavior problems in children who've never had them. CBS 2 Medical Editor Mary Ann Childers reports there's new research parents need to know about some hyper ingredients.*
>
> *In preschool, 3-year-old Cody Davis was in constant motion. He*

was hyperactive, aggressive and a trouble-maker.

"One time they called me and just said he's hurting other kids at school just because he's so wild, he can't control himself," said Cody's mother, Sheri Davis.

On the Internet, Davis stumbled on something she didn't expect: a link between behavior and food dyes.

"And that's when I started looking at what he was eating," she said.

Now, a highly regarded British study says a variety of common food additives -- including yellow dyes 5 and 6 -- can make kids hyper. And the findings are not just in children who have been diagnosed with attention-deficit hyperactivity disorder. In the study, most of the 300 children exposed to artificial colorings had some increased level of hyperactivity.

"It may impact actually the general population, not just ADHD persons, but the average child," said Dr. Thomas Blondis, M.D. of the pediatrics department at the University of Chicago's Comer Children's Hospital.

The link between additives and behavior was first made in the 1960's by an allergist named Dr. Benjamin Feingold. He developed a diet that many families use and many doctors recommend to this day.

"It's really just a difference of brands that you're buying," Davis

said. "For everything that you would normally eat, there's always a different brand that doesn't have the dyes in it."

Davis believes Cody was especially affected by red dye #40, and when she eliminated it from his diet she noticed an almost immediate difference.

"Within two days hyperactivity was down 75 percent," she said. "It was just amazing, the difference."

The hyper ingredients are found in everything from beverages to baked goods. Davis shops now for more natural versions colored by fruit and vegetable extracts so Cody can still eat foods he loves -- even cheese curls.

Sugar, in moderation, is not a culprit for causing hyper behavior.

ADHD expert Dr. Mark Stein, Ph.D. says he thinks a hyperactivity reaction to food dyes is not that common, but it's not a bad idea to go for natural over artificial.

"You know, it certainly wouldn't harm a child to reduce food dyes, and pay attention to what they eat," Stein said.

Now age 7, Cody is winning awards for his excellent behavior in school.

This latest research prompted the British equivalent of the Food and Drug Administration to issue an advisory to parents that they should reduce foods with additives if they see changes in *their child's behavior.*

The FDA, which regulates additives in the U.S., has taken no action. However, the Center for Science in the Public Interest recommends that parents avoid food dyes, especially yellow 5 and 6.

© MMIX, CBS Broadcasting Inc.

Artificial Flavors

While many parents are aware of the impact of dyes, many do not realize that artificial flavors are just as bad. My kids react to artificial flavors just as much as dyes. There are very minimal restrictions on what companies can use to flavor a food. Artificial flavors are made from hundreds of different combinations of chemicals. Food manufacturers may start with a "natural" flavor, but in the end, there is nothing natural about it.

Vanillin is a popular artificial flavor. You'll find vanillin in many chocolates and in foods that are vanilla flavored. Real vanilla is expensive so they came up with their own artificial form that was much cheaper to make. Note that vanillin occurs naturally in the lignins (a compound found in plants) of vanilla beans. However, due to a discovery in the 1950's, some artificial vanillin is made from the waste products of paper mills. [14]

There are other ways to make vanillin as well. Some synthetic vanillin is made from guaiacol, which is a petrochemical, or petroleum. And then there's the Japanese woman who figured out how to make vanillin from cow dung! She even won an Ig Nobel Prize for it in 2007. She found that lignins could be extracted from cow manure that has been heated and pressurized for one hour. I know we should recycle, but this is ridiculous. [15]

Rest assured this vanillin is not approved for use in food. It is used in perfumes and other non-food items to produce a vanilla scent. But, it goes to show how far researchers are willing to go to come up with a cheap alternative to the real thing, and the kinds of things the government allows in our products.

What Are the Health Hazards of Artificial Flavors?

Since there are so many different chemicals used in artificial flavors, and companies do not even have to list each chemical they've used, it is hard to test each and every one for ill side effects. Below is a small sampling of what we do know.

"Borneol is an artificial flavoring that may cause gastrointestinal irritation, seizures, confusion, and dizziness. Butryic acid has caused cancer in lab animals. Butyl acetate, a related chemical, can be toxic in high quantities. Carvacrol is an artificial flavoring that can lead to respiratory and circulatory depression as well as cardiac failure. Cinnamyl formate or formic acid, which is artificial cinnamon, has caused cancer in mice and may affect our kidneys." [16]

Some food critics say to avoid both artificial and natural flavors. Some natural flavors are derived from truly natural ingredients and some are not. The Feingold Association researches this. Food manufacturers are given a lot of liberty in using the term "natural flavors."

"The term natural flavor or natural flavoring means the essential oil, oleoresin, essence or extractive, protein hydrolysate, distillate, or any product of roasting, heating or enzymolysis, which contains the flavoring constituents derived from a spice, fruit or fruit juice, vegetable or vegetable juice, edible yeast, herb, bark, bud, root, leaf or similar plant material, meat, seafood, poultry, eggs, dairy products, or fermentation products thereof, whose significant function in food is flavoring rather than nutritional." [17]

This definition gives food manufacturers a lot of room to add just about whatever they want and call it a natural flavor. MSG is often hidden in natural flavors as are preservatives like BHA and BHT. If I see natural flavors listed on a product, I make sure to check my Feingold shopping guide to see if it truly is natural.

What About Preservatives?

Preservatives are just as problematic as dyes and artificial flavors. Some are made from petroleum as well. Before writing this book, I didn't know very much about the dangers of preservatives. I just knew that Feingold said they were bad and caused an adverse reaction in my kids. That was enough for me. We avoided them.

The preservatives avoided on Feingold are BHA, BHT, and TBHQ. They are sometimes listed as antioxidants because they keep food, particularly oils and fats, from going rancid. A chef I know said she wouldn't feed this stuff to her dogs - and rightly so. Researchers have done studies on feeding BHT and BHA to animals and here is what one researcher had to say.

In an article entitled, "The Saga of BHT and BHA in Life Extension Myths", Dr. JG Llaurado states: "…information in the bio-medical literature reveals that the recommended human dose of two grams per day is simply one order of magnitude below the lethal dose in animals.

Obviously, these high dose levels, if not immediately lethal for humans, must produce pathological effects." [18]

Sharla Race wrote a PDF book entitled *Antioxidants: The Truth About BHA, BHT, TBHQ and Other Antioxidants Used As Food Additives.* Here is a quote from the book: "A leading manufacturer of BHA has the following caution on its product specification. "Warning! Possible cancer hazard. May cause cancer based on animal data. Risk of cancer depends on duration and level of exposure. Harmful if swallowed. Irritant. Causes eye, skin and respiratory tract infection." [19]

The health issues associated with BHT, BHA, and TBHQ are many including headache, stomach issues, skin irritation, ADHD symptoms, eye irritation, tumors, asthma, and lung irritation. Pregnant mice that were given doses of these preservatives had offspring that slept less, were more irritable, and showed slower learning. [19]

BHA gives me a headache. I was buying some GFCF cupcakes from the health food store that were made at a local bakery. The ingredients read clean but every time I ate them, I got a headache the following day. I decided to contact the manufacturer to find out if the cupcakes contained any unacceptable ingredients. Sure enough, they use oil that contains BHA to spray their pans, which was not listed on their ingredients. No more cupcakes for me.

BHA and BHT were originally developed to serve as a preservative for petroleum. In the 1950's, BHA and BHT were approved for use in food. [19] The preservatives are mostly used to preserve fats and oils but are also used in cosmetics, toiletries, and medicines. It is best to buy cold pressed oils to try to avoid these preservatives.

In a December, 2011 article entitled, ""For Added Freshness" Label Claim Really Means "Added Chemicals" When It Comes to BHA and BHT," D. Wells from Natural News reported, "BHT is banned in England because research shows it reacts with other ingested substances to cause the formation of carcinogens. BHA is listed as a carcinogen by the state of California because it causes cancer in humans. BHA has been banned in Japan because studies found it causes cancerous tumors in rats' stomachs. Both BHA and BHT are toxic to the liver and kidneys. Remember, humans are animals too. Human lymph nodes absorb these toxins, and that's why breast cancer numbers have gone through the roof." [20]

TBHQ was approved for use in food in the early 2000's and is a chemical that is derived from petroleum and is a form of butane. [20] It was a sad day in our house when Feingold announced Eggo Buttermilk waffles which were once approved were adding TBHQ. We went out and found all the remaining Eggos we could find that still had the old ingredients.

TBHQ is being used more and more since states started putting bans on trans-fats. [21] In order to preserve the foods and extend the shelf life, manufacturers are often using TBHQ instead. Many restaurants like McDonald's are cooking their fries and chicken nuggets in oil preserved with TBHQ. [21]

Industrial workers exposed to the vapors of TBHQ suffered clouding of the eye lens. [19]

In February, 2011, in an article entitled, "TBHQ: Why This Preservative Should Be Avoided", Shona Botes from Natural News reported: "Consuming high doses (between 1 and 4 grams) of TBHQ can cause nausea, delirium, collapse, tinnitus (ringing in the ears), and vomiting. There are also suggestions that it may lead to hyperactivity in children as well as asthma, rhinitis and dermatitis. It may also further aggravate ADHD symptoms and cause restlessness. Long term, high doses of TBHQ in laboratory animals have shown a tendency for them to develop cancerous precursors in their stomachs, as well as cause DNA damage to them." [22]

Some people will argue that a person would have to eat a large amount of these preservatives in order to cause some of these more severe symptoms. I agree. However, what happens when a small, developing child or toddler consumes these preservatives? Many Feingold members report that TBHQ causes their kids to become extremely angry, crabby, or weepy.

What happens when they consume these preservatives daily, over the course of 30, 40, or 50 years? Studies have already shown that TBHQ is a carcinogen. Why would I want to chance this on my child when there are other food options available that do not use TBHQ as a preservative?

Why would some food manufacturers use TBHQ and others not? In my opinion, I believe it comes down to money. For example, if a food manufacturer uses TBHQ, maybe they would get three years shelf life out of their product. If they do not use TBHQ, they would either have to use another more natural preservative that is more costly, or they would forfeit the shelf life of their product, making it only good for perhaps one year instead of three.

If they don't sell all of their products within one year from production, they would have to discard all of them. And if consumers don't know manufacturers are using a dangerous chemical to preserve their food, or no one makes an issue out of it, they're going to continue to use it so they can make more of a profit.

This is where we as consumers come in. Tell manufacturers you don't want them using dangerous chemicals in your food. Or, stop buying foods with chemicals and urge your family and friends to do the same. Eventually, the drop in sales will affect their bottom line, and manufacturers will be forced to make better products. We are already seeing this happening with some products which is awesome.

If I have piqued your interest in removing these harmful chemicals from your family's diet, keep reading. I'll tell you why and how we started the Feingold Diet and how you can avoid all these harmful additives.

Chapter 3

Changes We Saw

We officially started the diet the first week in February. Within two to three days, my son was a completely different child. Hyperactivity went down about 75 percent. He was more focused and attentive. He was actually pleasant to be around. It seemed like everything I had tried to implement from the discipline books I had read, he suddenly responded to in the way he was supposed to. He *had* heard me (and he heard it often). He *could* obey!

Before Feingold, my son was always running everywhere, fidgeting, and talking non-stop. He couldn't look me in the eye because he was constantly in motion. Suddenly, he was calm. He started making eye contact, stopped fidgeting, and stopped running everywhere! Hallelujah!

He knew what was expected of him, and when he would get silly, he could quickly regain composure if I asked him to - something he could never do before. I always felt like he had wanted to obey me, but he couldn't. I could see the remorse in his eyes when he got in trouble before. Now it made sense. When he was eating those chemicals every day, he lost a lot of his self-control.

I remember shortly after starting the diet feeling extremely guilty and sad. I was grieved thinking that the first four years of his life could have been so much better. I had spent it spanking and scolding him, trying to get him to behave, and beating myself up thinking I was a terrible parent. The change in diet made it obvious that to some degree, he couldn't help it. As soon as we removed the offending foods, he was eager to please us. I found myself no longer yelling at him all the time to behave. Our house was so much more peaceful.

He was happy to do the diet because he wasn't getting into trouble anymore. He no longer became hyper from candy like before. It wasn't all about the sugar after all as so many people were telling me. Yes, sugar isn't healthy and should be used in moderation. It can cause yeast overgrowth, short term hyperactivity, and other health issues. The difference is, with dyes, the hyperactivity or "sugar high" doesn't last a couple of hours. It can last a couple of days. If they are eating chemicals every day, then it becomes a constant state of hyperactivity.

Hypersensitivity to Light Disappeared

Two months into the diet, my son's hypersensitivity to light suddenly disappeared. This was a child who would not go outside without a hat on - ever. He hated the sun in his eyes. He always cried as a baby in the car. I was hyper aware of when the sun was going down and I avoided going out in the car with him at that time.

We always kept a hat, sunglasses, and an umbrella in the car for him to block the sun. He would scream and cry about the sun being in his eyes. A holistic doctor told me he was hypersensitive to light. I didn't know there was such a thing.

One day in the car, before starting Feingold, he started screaming and crying frantically, like he was in great pain. He screamed that the sun was in his eyes. I had to pull the car over to get him to calm down because he was so distraught. I later bought a van with tinted windows to help with his issues with the sun.

After starting the diet, he suddenly stopped needing to wear a hat outside all the time, and stopped complaining about the sun being in his eyes. I was amazed! Apparently, this is not uncommon. Many ADHD kids and kids on the autism spectrum have hypersensitivities of the senses - sight, sound, smell, and touch. The official name for it is Sensory Processing Disorder (SPD). [1] My son also had a lot of noise sensitivity issues as a young child. He screamed and covered his ears when I ran the vacuum cleaner (lucky for him, it wasn't that often).

When you remove things that are offensive to the body like food additives, sometimes sensitivities suddenly improve. My son also went through a stage where he hated tags on his clothes. It drove him crazy. We had to cut all of the tags out of his shirts. The immune system can misinterpret normal occurrences like sight, sounds, and touch, and overreact to them.

For my son, it was obvious that the dyes and chemicals (and possibly salicylates) were the cause of his SPD symptoms because when we removed them, many of his sensory issues instantly disappeared. In talking with other Feingold members, I discovered there were other kids that had the same issues before starting the diet.

For some kids, hypersensitivity or SPD can be caused by foods like gluten or dairy, or whatever their bodies have misinterpreted as an invader. For other kids, the cause of their SPD symptoms is still unknown.

To this day (at age 13), my son will have hypersensitivity to light if he eats off diet. If he eats off diet, it's usually on the weekend. On Sunday, he will not be able to sit in church because of the lights. His eyes water and he buries his head in his lap because the light hurts his eyes so much. He usually gets up and waits in the lobby. Any other day when he is eating clean, the lights do not bother his eyes at all.

What About Detox?

When you start reading on the Feingold Facebook groups (see List of Resources at the end of this book), you will sometimes come across the subject of detox. Detox is the undesirable side-effects from starting the diet because of the body ridding itself of the toxins from the chemicals they were eating. Side-effects are usually mild (I sound like a commercial for drugs). We did not see any and many people don't. Occasionally someone might see their child acting up first before they start to see improvements. This should not last for more than a few days or weeks (if that long).

A week or so after starting the diet, my son was coloring with markers and got marker on his neck. He immediately broke out in hives, starting on his neck which quickly spread to his face, stomach, and legs. He had never had hives before in his life. They went away in a couple of hours but I guess he was reacting to the dyes in the marker.

That was the only time this happened. I think his body was detoxing so when he came into contact with the dyes, he had a strong reaction to it. He later would get marker on his hands at school and never had a reaction (but we tried our best to avoid any kind of ink on the skin).

Improvements in School

As I described earlier, my son's preschool teachers told me they saw red flags for ADHD - inability to sit still and concentrate. His report cards were always excellent on the academic portion, but the behavior section was awful.

After starting the Feingold Diet, I decided to homeschool him for kindergarten. I loved homeschooling and so did he for the most part. I couldn't believe how easy it was to teach him and how much I enjoyed spending time with him. Before starting Feingold, I would have never attempted homeschooling because I would have wanted the break that school gave me. By second semester, we could afford a Christian school and my son really wanted to go to be with other kids. He is an extrovert by every definition and is energized by being with other people.

So, we enrolled him in a Christian school. I wasn't sure what to expect as this was the first full year of being on the Feingold Diet in school. However, when we got his report card, he had no bad marks for behavior. His entire report card was excellent! I mentioned to his teacher that his preschool teachers told me they thought he may have ADHD. She looked at me bewildered and said she saw NO signs of ADHD.

By first grade, he was receiving awards - Excellence in Social Habits and Excellence in Work Habits. To receive these awards, the kids had to show consistent good habits in areas such as relating well to peers, using time wisely, and the like. He was also given the Diligence Award for always working with all of his heart. He won the first grade spelling bee and consistently gets comments like "A pleasure to have in class!" year after year on his report cards. We never would have seen comments like that before Feingold. We just laughed. I wanted to frame them!

In first grade, the kids would have to flip a card if they were misbehaving or talking. My son only got flipped a couple of times the entire year. Many kids got flipped nearly every day. He would tell the teacher that kids were misbehaving because of the dyes they were eating. He would come home and beg me to let him talk to the moms of the kids in his class. He said he would stand at the door during dismissal and tell them about Feingold. He wanted to make little business cards about the Feingold Diet and hand them out. Today, in eighth grade, he continues to get A's and B's and compliments from teachers on his report card. Going in to high school at a private school next year, he will be taking mostly honors classes.

Social Improvements

Family parties used to be a huge stressor for me. We would often leave early just because my son was acting up. After starting the diet, as we were leaving the party (and not early this time), a relative stopped me. She asked in amazement, "He's so much calmer. What did you do?" Of course I told her about Feingold.

Another day we went to visit our old neighbor. We moved before starting Feingold so she had not seen him since he started the diet. She had babysat my son for a couple of years (during his wild days). As I was talking to her, she looked at my son and looked concerned. She said, "Is he sick?" I said, "No, why?" She said, "He's just so quiet." (and calm).

Before Feingold, he was in constant motion, talking incessantly. He probably would have interrupted my conversation several times by then. You might think that Feingold may change your child's personality. It doesn't. My son was still the same talkative, lively little boy, but now he was in control of himself. He wasn't as impulsive and out of control. This was a welcome change.

When playing with neighbors before the diet, my son was often aggressive and argumentative. Most of the time, I had kids play at our house so I could keep an eye on him. One day, just days after starting the diet, my son went to our neighbor's house to play. My neighbor knew that we had just started the diet, and she told me she really noticed a difference in his behavior. She said the kids were playing play dough, and instead of fighting over everything like usual, they were playing very nicely! She didn't have to step in once. She was shocked.

Overall the improvements we saw were: hyperactivity went down *big* time, ability to control himself improved greatly (no more touching other kids constantly and sitting too close), he listened much better and followed through on what was asked of him (before it was like talking to a moving wall), hypersensitivity to light disappeared overnight, he stopped constantly fidgeting, he started to make eye contact when I talked to him (never did before), his tics stopped (when we removed all salicylates), his illness rate went down about 75 percent, he started making more friends, tantrums, crabbiness, and mood swings decreased dramatically (once we removed chocolate and corn syrup as well), he was less argumentative, he was much quieter (pre-Feingold, he would talk non-stop or make weird noises) and he was just so much more pleasant to be around. I felt like I had taken off a mask that had kept me from seeing my son for who he truly was. We were so thankful to have found the Feingold program!

Chapter 4

How We Started the Diet

Once I signed up for the membership, I e-mailed Feingold and requested the log in name and password for the association's web site. I couldn't wait to get on the member's message board to read and ask questions. (Now you can go on to Facebook and start reading and chatting there too. See "List of Good Resources" at the end of this book.)

I got some ideas on getting started and I slowly emptied my pantry shelves. I wasn't sure if I should use up the food I had or just get rid of it. I watched my son for reactions if he ate any unapproved foods. I quickly decided that I didn't want to feed him foods that I knew were bad for him, even though it meant wasting money on food that was already paid for.

Out With the Old. In With the New.

We had shelves full of Kraft macaroni and cheese, SpaghettiOs, Campbell's soup, and Pop Tarts. Everything a typical American kid eats, or basically, everything you see on cartoon commercials. Oh, and the "fruit" snacks of course. I thought these were good for him because the packaging said it contained lots of Vitamin C and even contained a full serving of fruit. I thought he was getting food from all of the five food groups so we were doing good, right?

I gave all the unapproved food to an extended family member who was struggling financially. She greatly appreciated it so I didn't feel as bad wasting all that money and I figured her kids were eating this stuff anyway. Sometimes people feel bad giving away food they know is bad, but I figure everyone needs to come to that place for themselves. Not giving them the food wasn't going to change how they ate so I didn't worry about it. You could also donate the food to a local food pantry.

I managed as best I could until our Feingold materials arrived. I read all I could on the Feingold message board. I tried to stick to the basics like meat, chicken, potatoes, and veggies and steered clear of any dyes. Some people choose to use up the food they already have and then start the diet after that. It's a personal choice.

Did We Start Out Doing the Diet 100 Percent?

Not completely. It took me a couple weeks to read through all the materials and understand the diet. Meanwhile, my kids had to eat. Our Whole Foods was about forty minutes away so I was only making a trip there once or twice a month.

I had to figure out which stores carried the foods I was looking for. Then I had to locate those foods within those stores. It was not easy to start the diet. Someone compared starting the diet to learning to drive a car for the first time. It's scary and overwhelming at first, but within a few months of driving, you no longer even think about it anymore. You just get in and drive.

The most challenging part of the diet is probably finding the food. Feingold lists out the approved foods, but they don't tell you where to find them. I needed more organization. Using the shopping guide, I made my own personal shopping lists by store. I listed some of these on my web site, and am starting to put lists together on my Pinterest page. Just be aware that some of these items may be outdated and no longer accepted or are not officially accepted but that we use without a problem. As well, there are many more accepted products that we just don't use. Newbies should stick to the Feingold shopping guide at first.

When you first go shopping for your Feingold-accepted foods, leave the kids at home. I was very overwhelmed at first. I was looking for foods that I wasn't sure were even there or what they looked like. That's why I love Whole Foods. Most of their foods are acceptable on the Feingold Diet (but not all).

When we first started the diet, there were these character graham cracker cookies that my son loved. They weren't Feingold-accepted but when I read the label, it looked like it *only* contained artificial flavors. I knew that dyes were bad and I wanted to avoid those, but I wasn't convinced about artificial flavors yet. So, I let him eat them sometimes. As we started the diet and he started to calm down, I started to notice that he did react to those artificial flavors and I finally bought into the whole diet, not just the avoidance of dyes.

As for stage one of the Feingold Diet, I wasn't completely convinced of that either. I hated telling him he could not have fruit. It just didn't seem American. We've all been raised to believe that fruit is good for you, and it is. However, the salicylates can be a big problem for some kids. I'll discuss salicylates in the next chapter.

In the first few weeks of the diet, I decided to let him still have his nightly snack of apple slices. I remember posting on the Feingold message board and asking if it was really necessary to do stage one completely. I explained how my son still had some issues, but that he was eating apples every day. They explained that I couldn't expect success if I was only trying the program halfway. I decided to pull the apples, and did notice that my son indeed had issues with apples. Thus began our journey of doing the Feingold Diet, stage one and 100 percent compliance with the diet.

How I Got My Son to Do the Diet

How did I convince my son to start the diet? Well, he was four and I was Mom. He was going to eat what I gave him. Okay, it was a little more than that, but for the most part, he went along with it and I was very grateful. If you have older kids, you might run up against more resistance, and have to deal with cheating when they are away from home. I'll address that later in this chapter, but for us, it was pretty easy to get my son's cooperation.

I explained to him why we were doing the diet. I told him what dyes were made of and that they were bad for him. I explained this further as he got older. I told him that dyes made it hard for him to control himself and that this diet was going to help him behave better. There was probably a better way to say that, but my son wasn't sensitive so I just told it to him like it was. He knew he got into trouble a lot. He recognized very quickly after starting the diet that he was better able to control himself.

Like many kids, I think he also enjoyed the extra attention he was getting. I was making new foods, just for him. I was shopping at new stores, just for him. I was ordering special candy online, just for him. He wasn't getting into trouble any more. He was staying out of time out. Mommy wasn't yelling anymore. Mommy was happy. He started to make friends at school, and they started asking him on play dates (first time ever).

It wasn't hard to convince him to do the diet. He was Feingold's biggest fan. He would tell family and friends that he was on "The Gold Diet." His favorite part was that he was able to eat ice cream and candy again.

I didn't know what it was in the candy and ice cream that made him so hyper (maybe sugar I thought), but I knew not to let him have any. When we started Feingold, I found approved ice cream and candy, and he didn't go off the wall. He would tell people all the things he avoided on the diet, but enthusiastically added, "But I can have sugar!" He was in heaven, and so was I.

Daddy's Food

I cleared the shelves of most of the unaccepted foods – at least those that were my son's favorites. There was no way I was going to leave one of his favorite foods sitting on the shelf for him to drool over, knowing he could not have it. One thing you can do is leave one top shelf for "Daddy's food" or fill in the blank. I explained to my son that people have different reactions or allergies to food. Some people can tolerate certain foods and other people cannot. I think teaching this concept to kids is important, especially today.

So many kids have allergies these days. Plus, I don't want my kids to judge other people for the way they choose to eat. I want them to understand that God created us all different and he gave us a free will to make choices for ourselves. I do tell them the truth though and when they get older I hope they will use good judgment in how they tell others about healthy eating.

I don't feel that God ever shames us or looks down on us, but instead is always loving and kind. Other parents can feel condemned or judged for how they feed their kids when they hear about Feingold. That's why I started my blog. Instead of pushing my views on others, if someone wants to learn more about the diet, they can read about it.

Some people like to say that they grew up eating all this food, and it hasn't affected them. Well, not yet anyway, and not in any way that they are aware of. Now that my kids are older, I've had to answer the question, "If dyes are bad, how come (fill in the blank) eats them?" I just have to explain that they *are* bad, and some people just choose to eat them anyway because they may not know any better or maybe they just don't care, but we are going to eat healthy out of reverence for God and His Word. For us it's partly a matter of personal conviction. I try not to push my personal convictions on others and I appreciate when others do not judge us for following our convictions.

Did I Put All of My Kids On the Diet?

At the time, I just had one other child, who was eighteen months old. I did not see any reason why not to put her on the diet too. I didn't want to make two different meals. She was very young when we started the diet and had no signs of hyperactivity. I didn't see Feingold as anything but a healthier way of eating for her. I did not make an effort to keep her on stage one though. She ate a lot of stage two fruits. I couldn't keep apple juice in the house though so I did switch her to pear juice and lemonade along with my son.

When she was about three, I started letting her have apple juice again. My son was well established on the diet and didn't get upset if someone else was having something he could not. I did notice that my daughter started having big meltdowns around this time. I thought it was from starting school and having a new baby in the house. I didn't link it to the apple juice till much later.

As a side note, I will say that initially your kids may want the same types of things that others are having. If at first, my daughter drank apple juice in front of her brother, he would whine and complain. After a while, it didn't bother him at all.

As another example, if other kids were having cotton candy, my son wanted cotton candy. (I did find an approved cotton candy online by the way and for a while, we made our own with a small cotton candy making machine). This will let up over time. Eventually, their favorite Feingold-approved candy, or homemade treat becomes better to them than anything the other kids are having.

Originally, I tried to sub everything as close as possible, including trying to match colors. Over time, my kids no longer cared if they got the same thing as other kids, as long as they got something good. They no longer cared if their cake was green. They discovered it tasted just as good with white frosting, and decorating it with natural green sprinkles or plastic figurines was just as much fun too.

Some people decide only to put their target child (the child you are initially doing the diet for) on Feingold because of cost concerns. They don't feel they can afford to buy Feingold-accepted foods for the whole family, or they have older children and don't feel that they would comply with the diet.

It's entirely up to you. Many families do for the most part eat Feingold-acceptable meals at home. Other family members may decide to eat off diet when they are away from home. Keep in mind that this whole diet is a learning process for everyone. While other members of the family may not be on board in the beginning, they may come around later, so don't give up hope.

Do I Do the Diet?

For the most part, yes, but I didn't do it 100 percent at first. I must admit, I ate horribly growing up. I feasted on fast food, pizza, doughnuts, and ice cream regularly. For some reason, I never gained weight. I was heavily involved in sports. I figured if I wasn't overweight, I was healthy.

The only thing I knew about food was what I learned in school - the five food groups. I thought I was doing well because pizza and McDonald's contained all the five food groups. French fries (potatoes) were my vegetable of choice.

When my son started the diet, I was forced to change my eating habits. I did not want to eat unacceptable foods in front of him. Plus, if I was asking my son to make these changes and lecturing him on the dangers of dyes, I thought I should be a good example and do the diet with him.

I did, however, keep my stash of Doritos hidden in the pantry in the beginning, but I would never let him see me eat them. I'm not saying it's wrong to eat unaccepted foods in front of your kids, but it wasn't something I chose to do.

Today, I do eat off diet every once in a while when I go out to eat or to a party. If my kids are with me and I decide to have the dessert, I make sure to eat it when my kids are not looking. Otherwise, I'll be asked, "Hey! Why do *you* get to eat that?" They're used to eating whatever I'm eating. I would say I do the diet at least 95% of the time.

My Own Detox

Feingold suggests avoiding fast food completely during stage one of the diet if you can. I avoided fast food as well by default because I didn't want to hear the whining from the backseat while I was going through the drive through.

After not eating fast food for six weeks and following the diet most of the time at home, I decided to get McDonald's for breakfast one day. The kids were not with me so I thought, "Hooray, McDonald's!" I got pancakes and sausage.

Soon after I got to work, I threw up. "I'm ruined!" I thought. What was going on? I had eaten McDonald's many times before without a problem. I think this was detox. My body had just spent the last six weeks cleaning itself out from all the junk I had been eating my whole life. When I fed it McDonald's, it did what it was supposed to do – expel the toxins and garbage. By the way, there are some Feingold accepted foods at McDonald's in Feingold's fast food guide. You just have to know which foods are OK there and which are not.

If you haven't seen the movie, "Super Size Me", you have to rent it from the library. This guy ate McDonald's every day for thirty days, at every meal. At first, he threw up from the food. Then, his body "adjusted". Of course, it led to a rapid decline in his health. He talks about food additives and all the junk that's in our food today.

Anyways, I was eventually able to eat out again but I tried to stick to Feingold-approved fast food. When I got pregnant with my third child, I did the diet 100 percent and I noticed quite a difference in my second son's behavior as a baby. He was much calmer than my older son, even though he was a boy! Imagine that. All boys weren't so bad after all! I continued the diet while nursing.

It wasn't until my fourth child that I really connected what I ate with my baby's behavior. I never paid much attention with my other kids. With my oldest, I knew if I had caffeine he was not going to sleep well that night and forget fast food. If I ate fast food (like burgers and fries), I was going to need a poncho because he would spit up like crazy.

With my fourth, I noticed that if I ate dyes or artificials, she was very fussy, fought going down for naps and would take a much shorter nap, waking up cranky. She was like this for about 36 hours. It was bad enough that I just stayed on the diet 100 percent. I did not want to deal with a fussy, sleepless baby for the next two days. It wasn't worth it. She otherwise slept extremely well and was a happy baby. She also rarely spat up. My oldest spit up constantly. The way my fourth child reacted when I ate off diet was the exact same way my oldest son was as a baby. I was eating dyes and artificials every day back then. Now I know why he was such a difficult baby.

I also noticed that when I eat something with artificial color or flavors, I have nightmares or really bizarre dreams that night. It's one of the ways I know when something has artificials in it or not. Feingold members have reported the same reactions.

Do Husbands Do the Diet?

Some husbands do and some do not. Some will eat clean at home, and then eat off diet at work. Do I think husbands would get big, big points with their wives if they did do the diet with the rest of the family (at least at home)? Yes. I think as leaders of the home, they would be setting a good example for their kids. They would be showing their kids the importance of practicing what you preach. In following the diet they are also showing support for their child. They are letting them know that they are important and worth making changes for, even though it might be hard.

I think it also shows love and respect to the wives, who are usually the ones at home, cooking and doing all they can to keep their child fully on the diet. At the very least, Dads should not frown upon the new meals their wives have made (it takes time to learn and try out new recipes). Dads, try to stay positive about the new changes and your kids will likely follow your example, and your wife will love you for it.

For me, it's just part of following God's commandment to love your neighbor as yourself. You certainly wouldn't wave beer in front of an alcoholic whom you loved, who just gave up drinking. So, if your child has to give up a favorite food, I say don't eat it right in front of them. Show them the same kind of love and respect that you would want to be shown.

I had a neighbor whose young kids had to start a gluten-and-dairy-free diet for serious health issues. She went out in the garage one afternoon to find her husband sitting eating his fast food in the garage. She told him he probably didn't need to do that (some kids are more sensitive than others). She thought it was really sweet of him to be so considerate of the kids though, and I did too!

How To Deal With Older Kids On the Diet

Many people starting the diet are doing so with younger kids, typically preschoolers. However, changes and improvements can be seen in anyone, at any age. If starting the diet with an older child, you may have some cooperation issues. It's easier to get a four- year-old to change their diet than a fourteen-year old. However, it's not impossible and it has been done.

For older kids, these harmful chemicals will affect them differently. They may not necessarily be hyper but they may have trouble concentrating and focusing in school. They may also have trouble controlling their anger, emotions, and moods. Educate your child on why the diet would be beneficial. They are old enough to understand. Let them do their own research as well. Watch some of the documentaries together that are listed at the end of this book.

If the child is on medication, explain that this is a possible alternative to the meds or a way to reduce them. There are some people who do both the Feingold Diet and medication, but some parents choose to wean their children off the medication after starting the diet because they see such great results, or they at least lower the doses of the medications they are on.

Talk to your doctor first before stopping any medication. Some doctors do not support the Feingold Diet, but there are a growing number who do. If a change in diet does work, it may suggest that many kids are unnecessarily prescribed ADHD medication every day.

I don't have any personal experience with ADHD medication but with any ailments or behavior issues, I personally prefer to seek out natural treatments first and resort to medication as a last resort when necessary. Though living with a child on the spectrum, there are some days where I have thought about it! But I'm reminded that many medications have unpleasant side effects, which send parents looking for alternative solutions such as the Feingold Diet.

I've heard from several parents whose kids started out on ADHD medication, only to then develop sleep issues, which led to medication for sleep. After that, the child developed emotional issues, which led to medication for depression. They sometimes also develop issues with their appetite. This is not uncommon apparently because I have heard from several parents telling me the same story of why they are now seeking an alternative to meds.

Medications are not the cure all and it is usually not a long term fix. With any medical issue, you really need to get to the root of the problem and find out what is causing the issues in the first place. For many kids, dyes and these other chemicals are the direct cause of their ADHD symptoms. It might be worth a try to remove the chemicals in their food first before trying medications.

Chapter 5

What Are Salicylates?

Salicylates are the natural chemicals that plants produce to ward off bugs and diseases. [1] Some fruits and vegetables produce more salicylates than others.

Dyes (or artificial colors) are a form of "salicylate radical." The most common reaction to radical salicylates (dyes) is hyperactivity and ADHD-like symptoms. Reactions from natural salicylates can be very similar to that of dyes. Often the kids that have strong reactions to dyes, will also react to salicylates, as they are both a form of salicylate.

Understanding Stage One and Stage Two

What is stage one and stage two of the Feingold Diet? Stage one is where you start for at least the first six to eight weeks. Before moving on to stage two, you need to see positive results or "success" for at least six to eight weeks. This may take longer than six to eight weeks for some kids. You will eliminate all high salicylate foods completely, while watching all moderate/medium and low salicylates. Salicylates can have a build-up affect so even eating too many low or medium salicylates can pose a problem.

After six to eight weeks of positive results, you can add back in stage two items one at a time and watch for reactions. Some people stay strictly stage one, but most people can add in at least some stage two foods in moderation after reaching baseline.

The foods eliminated in stage one are certain fruits, vegetables, nuts, and spices. The ones that we continued to eliminate because of obvious reactions were apples, grapes, and berries, and we do limited tomatoes. When my younger kids had even a small amount of these fruits they became very aggressive and had huge tantrums.

Below is a *partial* list of high, medium, and low salicylates. This is a list of the more common foods. For a complete list, see Feingold's handbook, which comes with a paid membership. A salicylate list is available on the Internet but it varies slightly from Feingold's list. I trust Feingold's list. It has been tested and found to be valid over and over by its members.

Low Salicylate

Fruit: Pears, lemons, limes, watermelon, honeydew, pomegranate, passion fruit, mango, kiwi, papaya, guava, etc.

Veggies: Asparagus, Brussels sprouts, broccoli, cauliflower, green beans, kale, lettuce, olives, onion, peas, sweet potato, carrots, pumpkin, parsley, etc.

Nuts: Cashews, pecans, sunflower seeds. Maple syrup and a long list of spices are also low salicylate.

Medium Salicylate

Fruit: Bananas, cantaloupe, avocado, canned pineapple (not fresh), grapefruit,

Veggies: White potato, spinach, etc.

Spices: Cinnamon, oregano, sage, cumin, and more.

Other: Honey (except for clover honey).

High Salicylate

Fruit: Apples, grapes, berries (including strawberries, blueberries, raspberries, etc.), cherries, apricots, grapes, raisins, nectarines, oranges, peaches, plum, prunes, tangerines, dates, fresh pineapple (note canned pineapple is a medium salicylate), etc.

Veggies: Cucumbers, pickles, peppers, tomatoes, zucchini, etc.

Spices: Cloves, oil of wintergreen, red pepper, paprika, chili powder, cayenne, rosemary, dill, ginger, and more.

Nuts: Almonds

Other: Molasses, clover honey

Tea and coffee are also high salicylate. [2]

You can eat freely from the low salicylates list, eat less frequently from the medium salicylates list, and test the high salicylates list (after completing stage one). Salicylates can have a build-up effect as well. Your child may not react right away from eating them, but if eaten frequently, they may suddenly have a build-up reaction a couple of days later. I know it sounds like a lot of foods to remove, but I will explain below why it is important to do stage one.

Feingold is very specific about what is stage one and stage two. The Feingold shopping guide is separated into two sections. If you are looking for an approved ice cream, you will go to the back to see what page ice cream is on. It might show page 73, 229. Page 73 will list the stage one approved ice creams, and page 229 will list the stage two approved ice creams. If you have the PDF version of the shopping guide, you can just do a search for the item you are looking for. On my phone, using Adobe Acrobat, I just have to hit an arrow to see the other stage.

Oh, No! Not the Apple Juice and Berries!

I think the biggest mistake people make when considering the Feingold Diet is that they don't understand the effect salicylates can have on their kids. When we first started the diet, I completely understood why to remove the dyes. It took me a little longer to come to grips with the artificial flavors and preservatives. But eliminating fruits? This I had a problem with. I thought, God gave us fruits and they are supposed to be good for us. Now I have to tell my child that he can't have apple juice and his favorite fruits?

The purpose of doing stage one is so you can get to that calm place, or baseline, and see how your child behaves without artificials, preservatives, and salicylates. When you have a child with behavior issues, it's easy to get accustomed to that non-stop action, hyper, whiny, aggressive, loud, boisterous child. It might not even faze you anymore because you have learned to live with it and just cope.

I had to talk myself into doing stage one for several weeks. I told myself it was only for a few weeks. We'd get through it. I told my son the same thing. I figured if we were going to do this diet, we might as well do it right. I didn't want to waste all our time and effort, doing the diet only partially, and only seeing partial results.

After the initial stage one of the diet, you can start to add back in stage two foods, one every few days. You should easily be able to see if a food is causing a problem or not.

Common Reactions to Salicylates

Here is a list of some common reactions to salicylates: Reddening of the ears or face, depression, moodiness, meanness, grouchiness, mood swings, irritability, chronic fatigue, mental and physical sluggishness, upset stomach, bladder incontinence, night wetting, eye muscle disorders, short attention span, inability to concentrate, poor self-image, fidgety, temper flare ups/tantrums, distractibility.[1]

On the Feingold boards, the reactions most often reported are tantrums, aggressiveness, and red ears. The most common culprits are apples, berries (especially strawberries), and grapes. Dark circles and bags under the eyes can also be caused by high salicylate foods. If dark circles are not eliminated from a low salicylate diet, they can also be caused by gluten and/or dairy.

How My Kids React to Salicylates

When my kids were little, I did not restrict the salicylates right away. I didn't think salicylates would be a problem. However, at church I was called to get my son out of the nursery two weeks in a row because he was fighting with other kids. I removed the high salicylate foods he was eating right before church and I never got called to the nursery again. In addition, he finally stopped his excessive biting habit.

My kids react to salicylates differently at different ages. Around the toddler years, my kids would bite, hit, and get very hyper and aggressive. My one son would bite up to fifty times a day before I discovered he was reacting to salicylates. I could not leave him alone for a second or he would be biting his siblings.

Around kindergarten, my kids get aggressive, hyper, and very whiny if they have too many salicylates. We don't eliminate salicylates completely, but do restrict them. One of my kids will have meltdowns from salicylates. Currently, my toddler does not seem to have too much of a problem with salicylates, other than occasional biting from eating too many.

Tourette Syndrome & Tics

Two of my kids have Tourette-like reactions or tics when they eat too many salicylates. [3] One year, one of my boys started chewing his shirt collars incessantly. He actually chewed holes through his shirts and wore out the collars of all his shirts. He would come home from school with a big wet ring around his collar every day. His teacher mentioned his chewing and I got him a chew necklace. That didn't help. She thought he might have anxiety. I didn't know what was causing these issues so I went online.

I learned that chewing (also called pica) can be a sign of zinc deficiency so we supplemented with zinc. [4] While I do believe he was deficient in zinc, supplementing with zinc did not stop his tics. Magnesium is another vitamin that can sometimes help reduce tics.[5]

Since supplementing didn't help, I started looking through the ingredients of the foods he was eating. As soon as school started, he started eating peanut butter breakfast bars almost every day before school, and occasionally had blueberries. I read the ingredients on the breakfast bars and noticed there were apples in them. I must have overlooked that when I bought them. I pulled them from his diet, and watched all other salicylates and he stopped chewing his shirts! Finally! He had chewed his clothes for about three or four months and instantly stopped. When I tested later to see if the apples and blueberries were causing his chewing, sure enough, when I gave him blueberries, he started chewing his shirt again.

In my research and in talking to other moms, I learned that tics can also be a symptom of yeast overgrowth (a big topic, to be explained in a future book). [6] All of the stage two fruits feed yeast. So, removing those fruits also removes those yeast feeders. I've noticed that one of my children experiences tics when they eat too much sugar as well. That supports my theory that yeast overgrowth and salicylate sensitivity are somehow related.

The tics my kids experience from salicylates change over time, as is common with Tourette Syndrome. My kids will have each tic for a few months and then all of sudden start doing something else from salicylates. I have no idea why this is. Sometimes my kids will cough habitually, clear their throat or blink really hard over and over. Sometimes they shrug their shoulders non-stop or stick their tongue out to the side. Sometimes they tap their pencil on the table or desk or open their mouth really wide. They don't even realize they are doing these things and it is out of their control. If I tell them to stop, they'll be doing it again a minute later.

My son went through a stage when he was about four where he could not stop snorting. Every five seconds or so, he would snort like a pig and couldn't stop. We were about to walk in to a school concert that had already started, and my son was snorting rather loud. We kept telling him to stop. He almost started crying and said, "I can't!" I took him outside for the remainder of the concert. We then pulled the fruits and watched the sugar intake, and he finally stopped snorting.

Day and Night Wetting

Salicylates can also cause day and night wetting. I discovered this when my daughter started the low oxalate diet (which is similar to Feingold stage one). When we started the GFCF diet (gluten-and-dairy free) when she was four, I let up on some of the stage one restrictions. It was about this time that she started having accidents after being completely potty trained for several months. Shortly after starting the GFCF diet, I decided to try a yeast free diet.

On a yeast free diet, blueberries and raspberries are allowed, but they are Feingold stage two fruits so we had been avoiding them. I started feeding them to her and she started having accidents at school and at home. She had not been dry at night yet so I didn't notice any change in that yet. She was too old to put in pull ups. I didn't know what to do. I started doing some research and discovered that many of my daughter's symptoms were symptoms of high oxalates in the body. [7]

We started her on the low oxalate diet, which eliminates many of the same fruits eliminated in Feingold stage one. There are a few fruits that are high salicylates and low oxalate, like apples. We tried apples for a while, but those proved fatal - major tantrums. When we stuck to a low salicylate and low oxalate diet, she was noticeably calmer, she immediately stopped having accidents, and for the first time in her life, she woke up dry several days in a row. She also stopped having frequent urgent trips to the bathroom and severe eye pain, which are other signs of elevated oxalates in the body.

If you think oxalates might be an issue, the yahoo group, "Trying Low Oxalates" is a good place to start to learn more. [8] I also did a post on the Low Oxalate Diet on my web site. [9] The Low Oxalate Diet is sometimes helpful for kids with autism as yeast overgrowth and high oxalates often coexist.

If your kids have issues with wetting, it could be caused by other things too. Yeast overgrowth can also cause wetting issues, but again, avoiding stage two fruits also means you are avoiding yeast feeding fruits too.

Wetting can also be caused by a food intolerance like dairy or some other food. The best way to figure that out is to keep a diet diary and log when they are having accidents, if it's not every day. I have a hard time believing any doctor that says wetting is caused by anxiety or is a behavior issue. What kid wants to have an accident? Supplementing with magnesium can also help as it will help the bladder muscles stretch. [10]

Does Everyone Need to Do Stage One?

If you are doing the diet for a child with ADHD or other behavioral issues, I would say you definitely need to do stage one. If you are doing the diet for other family members who just want to avoid harmful additives and eat healthier, I think it's perfectly fine to skip stage one. You may later discover that your family does react to salicylates and decide to remove them at a later time. There are some kids who do not react to salicylates and I see no problem with them continuing to eat high salicylate foods.

Is Stage One Forever?

In general, the longer you eat a clean diet, the less reaction you should have to foods. The body needs time to heal and clean itself out so it can handle the occasional "offensive" food or environmental trigger (strong scents like perfumes, etc.) properly. For some kids, this can take a long time, and they may need to stay on stage one for a while. And then there are some kids who can go straight into stage two after just six weeks. It really varies but I would say that most kids with ADHD end up staying mostly stage one, being able to handle some stage two in moderation. That's what we do.

If salicylates didn't cause such a problem, I would certainly let my kids indulge. We limit stage two more during the school year than in the summer, which works out nice because more of the stage two fruits are in season in the summer.

We try to reserve stage two foods for special occasions and vacations, or the weekends. I'm not going to give my child grapes right before a school concert. If we're on vacation, I'm more inclined to let my kids have stage two fruits, and I just brace myself for the possible reaction. I like at least knowing why my kids are reacting and how to avoid a reaction.

While my kids react to both the harmful chemical additives and natural salicylates, my bigger issue is obviously with the harmful additives. I'm not going to let my kids have dyes just because it's summer and they're not in school.

After completing stage one (seeing positive results for at least six to eight weeks), it's really up to you if you want to stay stage one or move to stage two. You have to see how much salicylates affect your child and how much you are willing to tolerate. If your child just gets red ears, maybe you can live with that. If they are having problems at school from eating salicylates, then obviously you would probably want to stay mostly stage one.

For kids with autism, as reported by many parents on the message boards, stage two foods can often cause meltdowns and aggression. My daughter was never hyper. When we started the diet when she was eighteen months old I never thought to keep her strictly stage one. I later saw how very much she reacts to stage two foods.

What About Ketchup and Tomatoes?

Ketchup and tomatoes are probably the hardest things to avoid in stage one. I was extremely lucky in that my son hates ketchup and anything with tomato sauce. He eats his noodles plain or with parmesan cheese. Some kids eat noodles with butter or with a homemade Alfredo sauce. My son likes his pizza with extra cheese and no sauce. I have a recipe for a garlic sauce at the end of the book that you can dip pizza in. You can tell your kids you're having garlic bread with cheese.

Feingold has an un-tomato spaghetti sauce, un-tomato ketchup, and an un-tomato pizza sauce recipe that uses stage one ingredients like beets but I've never tried them since my son doesn't like tomato products anyway. Some people like the un-tomato recipes and some hate them. Most people just try to avoid ketchup. In my opinion, I would try to reduce the ketchup as much as possible by choosing meals that don't typically need ketchup. That requires some creativity but it's not impossible.

For me, avoiding the artificial flavors, colors, and preservatives are my first priority. If my kids have some ketchup, I don't flip out over it, but

I do realize that they might react from the tomatoes. In our house, we just try to reduce the amount of tomato products we eat, and try to keep it to the weekends. If you are eating out, almost all of the ketchup contains corn syrup (may be listed as dextrose). I try to bring our own ketchup if we go out because we personally avoid corn syrup.

I put some in a small Tupperware container or I even have some of the little plastic disposable three-ounce containers that restaurants use that I ordered on Amazon. Whole Foods sometimes has the Simply Heinz brand ketchup in packets at their restaurant. These do not contain corn syrup. I keep our extra packets in the car.

Am I saying you should cheat and allow some stage two products such as ketchup during stage one? No. I'm saying you should try to avoid all stage two products during stage one, but if cutting out ketchup makes it too hard for you to keep your kids on the diet at all, I'd rather see someone give in on the ketchup issue then to give up on the whole diet completely.

Yes, your kids may react from the ketchup, and unsupportive relatives or teachers may say that the diet doesn't work. But, for me personally, I'm at peace knowing that I am feeding my kids food that is not causing them physical harm or behavioral issues. My focus is my child's overall health, not just avoiding a reaction. At some point, I just developed a tougher skin and stopped letting the comments or opinions of others affect me and how I fed my children.

Chapter 6

Grocery Shopping

Grocery shopping for the first time when starting the diet is going to be overwhelming. Leave the kids at home. When you get your food guide, go through it and highlight or underline items you think your kids might like and then make a list. Don't forget that you can also stick to the basics like meats, chicken, and produce. The hardest part of grocery shopping is not knowing what these products look like, and which stores to find them in. There are some items you are only going to find in Whole Foods or a health food store, and other items that you will have to locate in your regular grocery store.

Don't panic. This problem is only temporary. Once you find the products your kids like, and find where you can buy them, you will just go into repeat mode. And don't forget that you can post on the Feingold Facebook group and ask for help.

I have a post on my web site with pictures of the foods I bought from which stores over a 30-day period.[1] I also posted a grocery list that I made for my family when I was expecting a baby. [2] While not all of the foods are in the shopping guide (there are some companies that will not work with Feingold but that read clean and we eat without a problem), and some of the foods are no longer approved, it will give you a general idea of the kinds of foods you can buy where.

Feingold also has a few links on their web site and on their Facebook group of sample grocery lists by store. For example, someone posted what they typically buy from Sam's Club and Costco. This can be helpful to use as well. I've started using Pinterest so I can let my family see pictures of the foods that my kids can eat when they are in their care. Some other Feingold members have done this as well. This might be a good place for you to keep track of foods that each of your kids like, and an easy way to keep your husband in the loop of acceptable foods.

What If I Don't Have a Whole Foods Store Near Me?

I hear this question a lot. Whole Foods is Feingold heaven. Many of the foods are Feingold acceptable - not all, but a lot of it is. My kids love going to Whole Foods with me because they know they get to load up the cart with lots of good stuff - that and the fact that they have an awesome natural bakery and restaurant. Well worth the trip if you have to drive a little farther to get to one.

Our Whole Foods now is about twenty-five minutes away which isn't bad. I go there about once a month. Some people drive two hours with a big cooler every few months. If you do live far, they provide free bags of crushed ice to put in your grocery bags if you ask, and be sure to bring insulated bags for your frozen foods.

Whole Foods can be expensive. My brother likes to call it "Whole Paycheck." However, you can also get a lot of good deals on occasion. Visit Whole Foods' web site before you head out and print out any coupons you might need. There is no limit on the number of coupons you can print out online. Their coupons change about once a month or two. They have coupon booklets up front near the front doors or near customer service with more coupons in them. I've scored some really good deals (even free food) by doubling manufacturer coupons with Whole Foods' coupons.

There are some foods that I can only find at Whole Foods but that's been improving as more stores are carrying the more natural foods now. 365 Brand is the brand name for the store so of course those will only be found at a Whole Foods. While many things at Whole Foods are clean, you can't depend on Whole Foods to weed out all the bad stuff. They are not checking with all the food manufacturers to find out what exactly is in all the food they are selling. If you buy something from the bakery, you might need to double check to make sure they are not using a spray with BHT on the bakery pans. In most cases, they do not.

There are also some other smaller franchises that carry a lot of the same foods Whole Foods carries. In the Midwest we have Mariano's, Woodman's, and The Fresh Market.

Find a Health Food Store

If you don't have a Whole Foods near you, you have my condolences. However, it's not necessary in order to do Feingold. It just makes life a little easier and more convenient. Most areas of the country will have a health food store. You may not even know you had one near you. They will have a similar selection as Whole Foods, but on a smaller scale. There are some bigger health food stores that are part of a chain of stores. Those will typically have better prices than an independent health food store. Near Chicago we have Fruitful Yield health food stores. In Orlando they have Chamberlin's.

If there is something you want that your health food store doesn't have, ask if they can order it for you. Some stores will make you order a whole case if they order it though. Talk to the store and see what they can do for you. If they know you are going to be coming in and purchasing from them, they may be happy to work with you. I had my health food store order me a case of Rudi's bread. After that, they decided to start carrying the bread.

Order Online

Once you find a food that you know your child likes, see if you can order it online. I order a lot of things on Amazon. I rarely pay shipping. You often have to buy at least $35 worth of something in order to get the free shipping though. I love that it comes right to my door. I often buy in larger quantities, but you can sometimes buy single items too if you just want to try it. Some of the products are the same cost as at the store so I figure why not have it delivered to my door?

What things do I typically buy online? I've bought cereal, snack type foods (popcorn, chocolate energy bars, breakfast bars), candy, gum, chicken broth, rice milk, diapers, shampoos, soaps, parchment paper, unbleached muffin cups, and a few other things. It takes a little time at first because I go online (usually to Amazon first) and check out the prices. Then I see if I can get it cheaper in the store. I also take into account if the item typically goes on sale or if coupons are ever available for that product.

Over time, you'll figure out where to purchase products for the best price and convenience. Some items I can only find online though. Personal care products like shampoo I can almost always find for much cheaper online. For those items, I typically purchase from www.vitacost.com, www.swansonvitamins.com, or www.iherb.com.

Trader Joe's

Trader Joe's is another store that contains a lot of Feingold acceptable foods. However, as of January, 2013, Trader Joe's stopped filling out forms for Feingold. They said their suppliers change ingredients so often that they don't feel confident that they are giving Feingold accurate information for the shopping guide. I like Trader Joe's for their organic produce and a few snack products.

Trader Joe's claims that their Trader Joe's brand name products contain no artificial colors, flavors, or preservatives. I've seen other brands of candy at their stores though that contain dyes so you have to read the labels. Feingold has never listed all of Trader Joe's foods as approved. One of the reasons is because not all of the products had been submitted for review before they stopped filling out forms. So, Trader Joe's is "eat at your own risk" and stick to the food guide if you are new to the diet. If you are not new to the diet, you can experiment with foods that read clean and see if your child reacts.

Your Local Grocery Store Has Options Too

While I'm not loading up my cart at my local grocery store chain, there are still some items that I get from there. Some grocery stores have a separate section for all of their organic, allergen free, and natural foods. I love that. I can go in and go to one section and have most of my grocery shopping done (partly because we are also gluten and dairy free). However, some of the stores I shop at have started to change that and incorporate all of the natural foods in with the regular stuff. I hate that. They want to lure you down every aisle so you make impulse buys.

There are some mainstream foods and basic staples that are approved. Check your Feingold shopping guide. I do most of my shopping at Woodman's (here in the Midwest) which has a nice two-aisle section with organic and natural foods, and their prices are better than Whole Foods. I go to my regular local grocery store (Meijer) for things like fresh produce, lemonade, and a few other items. Then I go to Whole Foods about once a month and stock up. I've noticed that I have not needed to go to Whole Foods as often as the mainstream grocery stores are starting to carry a lot more Feingold approved brands. I'm guessing this trend is going to continue, especially as more and more people start demanding better products.

Do I Have to Buy All Organic Food?

No. Organic food just tends to not contain artificial ingredients or preservatives, but not always. There are many foods in the shopping guide that are not organic. Some people like to buy organic to avoid GMO's (genetically modified organisms), and for other health reasons. Just because a food is labeled "organic" doesn't necessarily mean that 100% of the ingredients are organic. Some will even say, "Made with 70% Organic Ingredients."

And, not all "organic" or natural foods are going to be Feingold accepted. There are some that may use preservatives in their packaging. I'd like to think that makers of more natural or allergy friendly foods have higher ethical standards than the big food manufacturers, but that's not always the case.

Do I Need To Switch Out All Our Personal Care Items?

This is a question that you'll often stumble upon after purchasing the program. I know I was thinking, "Wait a minute, they're not eating the stuff. Why do I have to change shampoos and toothpaste?"

Not everyone switches these out right away. I think with all the changes in food, it's often something that is done a few weeks later after reading and taking it all in. I do think toothpaste is a good thing to change right away because kids' toothpaste is often brightly colored and flavored.

Anything that touches the skin is going to get absorbed. If you put lotion on, where does it go? It absorbs into the skin and gets into the bloodstream. I'm not vigilant about everything but when it is a simple change in brand, I don't see any reason not to switch them.

Below are some of the products we use. Approved brands can change their ingredients at any time, so please double check with your Feingold shopping guide before using these products for yourself if you are doing the diet.

For detergents, we have used Tide Free or Seventh Generation. We currently use a small amount of Seventh Generation and about ¼ cup of Borax because my daughter has very sensitive skin and breaks out from anything else. Many skin rashes and irritations are often caused by detergents. Many detergents contain perfumes which can be a problem for some kids. We don't use any dryer sheets because my daughter is too sensitive, but when we did, we used Bounce Unscented dryer sheets.

We use Ivory soap bars for the older kids and adults, and for babies, we use Rainbow Unscented shampoo and sometimes California Baby body wash and shampoo. California Baby is expensive and comes in a small bottle so I preferred to use the Rainbow for shampoo and then use the California Baby for the body wash. California Baby's conditioner didn't work well on my daughter's thick, curly hair. You can find these shampoos at Whole Foods or a health food store, but they are cheaper online. I often order through www.vitacost.com. Many baby shampoos contain dyes and other harmful chemicals.

Feingold doesn't have a big list of approved shampoos. I'm thinking they just haven't researched all of them. The ones we use are usually allergy free, without parabens or dyes, and are sometimes organic so my guess is that they are without all the bad chemicals too.

Currently we are using Mineral Fusion Curl Care for shampoo and conditioner - works very well on my daughter's curly hair. The Curl Care was the only one which had a light enough scent for us to tolerate. We use Desert Essence Unscented Body Wash for body wash. This doubles as bubble bath if you have a Jacuzzi tub. Trust me. We've used Desert Essence's Unscented shampoo and conditioner in the past as well but prefer Mineral Fusion for my daughter as their conditioner works better.

My daughter sometimes uses the raspberry scented Desert Essence shampoos though because she likes the smell. These are just the ones we use but they are not currently part of the Feingold shopping guide. I order these online or get them at my local health food store.

The kids use Tom's of Maine Silly Strawberry toothpaste. It is stage two, but it's the only toothpaste my kids like. They don't like anything minty. Most mainstream toothpastes are not approved because of dyes or artificial flavors. I use Desert Essence Tea Tree Oil and Neem toothpaste. I also like to avoid sodium laurel sulfate (SLS) and parabens in our personal care products if I can. The Tom's toothpastes do contain SLS. Tom's was bought out by Colgate. For mouthwash, The Natural Dentist and Tom's of Maine make an approved mouthwash.

What am I not vigilant about? Hand soap. I just get the big liquid hand soaps at Sam's Club. Anything that's white and without dyes listed. I know that just because it's white doesn't mean it doesn't contain chemicals, but that's what we use. I guess we could use Ivory soap bars in the bathroom and we did for a while, but I like using liquid soap. You can also make your own liquid hand soap, or some people use Dr. Bronner's soap. There are several recipes out there.

I don't use any colored or heavily scented soaps. Kids sometimes put their hands on their face while sitting at their desk at school and they are going to be inhaling that smell all day, and it can affect them. Perfumes give me a headache.

Schools tend to have soap that is scented and sometimes brightly colored. If your child is sensitive, you can send in your own approved soap bottle to only be used by your child. I did this when my son was in first grade. I told the teacher I wanted him to use that instead of the regular soap. They had a sink in the classroom for the kids to use after they did coloring or crafts. He had a really nice teacher that year, and she was happy to oblige.

If my kids go into a nursery or anywhere else where they want them to use hand sanitizer, I just tell them we have allergies and can't use that stuff. I don't have time to read the ingredients on what they want to put on my kids' hands, but for us, we avoid those because they are anti-bacterial and will kill ALL bacteria on the hands. This isn't good. We have good and bad bacteria on our hands and you don't want to kill both. Then your hands and skin are left unarmed when they come into contact with the bad bacteria again, which they will.

Read articles on www.mercola.com if you want to read more about anti-bacterial soaps and hand sanitizers. A lot of moms are religious about using hand sanitizer. I don't think they realize they are probably doing more harm than good. Some hand sanitizers contain alcohol too. Kids were licking their hands and ingesting alcohol and displaying drunk-like behavior. That's not good. They realized this, and have started taking alcohol out of some of these sanitizers. We just avoid hand sanitizers altogether and practice good hand washing instead.

Chapter 7

Where Do I Find Feingold Recipes?

You can find Feingold recipes anywhere. The Internet is my favorite place to look. www.allrecipes.com is one of my favorites. There are also hundreds of food blogs. There are too many to list my favorites. And then there's the library and of course Pinterest. You are just going to use Feingold approved ingredients. If you are stage one, make sure you are also using stage one ingredients. Feingold also has a Feingold Recipes Facebook group for Feingold members.

Tomatoes are my biggest challenge, as they are stage two. Tomatoes are in a lot of recipes that we might like. That can be a challenge. We just limit tomatoes since we are not strictly stage one. During stage one you should try to avoid all stage two foods if possible.

When we first started the diet, I didn't know where to start. I looked through the recipes on Feingold's Recipe Board, which you will have access to once you become a member. My mom cheerfully dropped off her huge collection of Taste of Home cookbooks and I started rummaging through them. Have your kids look through cookbooks as well. My kids loved doing this. They would excitedly tell me which foods they wanted me to make. Of course, they were mostly desserts.

When I found a recipe, I would look up the ingredients in the Feingold Shopping guide to make sure I got the right products. We tried new recipes and some of them were a fail. This was frustrating and time consuming, not to mention costly. But, I didn't give up. I tweaked recipes that didn't come out just right the first time, and tried again.

I remember making the marshmallow recipe in the Feingold Handbook three or four times before getting it right. Finally, I went on the message board and asked what the deal was. It's funny because nine years later, I still see the exact same question posted on Feingold's Facebook group every so often by newbies.

I found the answer to my question from some other Feingold moms. I was frustrated though. So the next time, I made the marshmallows, got it right, and wrote it all out. The recipe in the handbook does not specify that you need to beat the sugar mixture for about fifteen minutes. I was using a hand-held mixer and could not even imagine it would take fifteen minutes to get this stuff to thicken. My arms were killing me! I got a Kitchen Aide stand- alone mixer, and a candy thermometer, and finally, we had marshmallows! Yay! Happy dance. I could do anything now.

Eventually, I started typing out all the recipes that I got to turn out right and that were a success with my family. I wrote down exactly what I did, as I often needed more instruction than what was written on the recipe. I also included what Feingold accepted ingredients I used so that my mom or husband could make the recipe as well and so I wouldn't have to look up the approved ingredients again.

I checked out cookbooks from the library. I typed up the recipes I liked and made my own little personal cookbook. I put all the recipes in a three-ring binder with sheet protectors. This made my life in the kitchen much less stressful and more organized. It also saved me time.

I didn't have to search through the cookbooks to find the recipe I wanted.

I've posted the recipes we like on my recipe blog. I have them listed by stage one and stage two. I've also pinned them on to my Pinterest boards. Every family is different though and has different tastes based on ethnic origin or even what area of the country you live in. So, just look for recipes that are similar to what your family already likes and then tweak it to make it Feingold friendly.

At the end of this book, I've listed a few of our favorite stage one recipes to help you get started. I cook mostly GFCF now. My son is lamenting for the days when I made cinnamon rolls and soft pretzels. I am too! But, I can't make cinnamon rolls with my three younger ones in the house, drooling over them while they bake. So, he has to wait for Grandma to get back from Florida to make those for him.

Chapter 8

Is It Expensive?

Yes and no. If you buy a lot of natural, prepackaged, processed foods, you *are* going to pay more. However, I feel it is a trade-off. My grocery bills are higher, but my expenses for eating out are much less. We do use a lot of Ian's brand products which are costly as we are also GFCF, but I figure it still costs me less than eating out at a restaurant.

I take my kids to the doctor much less since starting the diet which saves me money. We save a whole lot by bringing our own food to places. Movies are one example. We make our own popcorn (we have a Whirly Pop style popcorn popper that I got online) and bring our own drinks to movies. I have four kids, so that would add up fast if we had to buy food. I put it all in a backpack and if they ever ask (they only have once); I just tell them my kids have allergies and can't eat any of the food they sell.

Had we not started the diet, I don't think I would have even thought to bring my own food places. It's really no big deal after you get used to it. Today, so many kids have allergies (partly due to the junk they are eating), that no one bats an eye anymore.

I save an enormous amount at places like Six Flags and Disney. I look at what my extended family is paying for their food and I'm so glad we are not paying that. I now make my own cakes for birthdays, which saves me about $20 per family member per year (which is more than the cost of a membership). Some people already make their own cakes or bring their own food places, but the average middle class family doesn't even think twice about it. It's those little things that add up.

You do not have to make all your food from scratch, but it will save you money, and it's healthier. I didn't start out making everything. I didn't know how to cook! My sister's favorite question was, "What's for dinner? SpaghettiOs or mac-n-cheese?" Ha, ha.

You learn. It won't happen all at once, but you will start making things that you never knew you could make and your kids will love it. Don't give up if you don't get it exactly right the first time. It usually takes me about three tries to get a recipe just right.

I also think of it this way, I'd much rather pay $69 (the current cost of the PDF) now, than be paying who knows how much later in life if heaven forbid my child comes down with some medical condition from eating so many harmful chemicals his whole life. Every parent would come up with the money to treat their child, no matter what the cost.

I see the Feingold Diet as a tool of prevention. It's normal to hear of people talk about how they watch what they eat now, because they've had cancer. Why not watch what you eat before you get cancer? I don't want to wait until that day to change the way my family eats. I want to teach my children when they are young how to eat properly so that they can have the best start in life and hopefully avoid many health risks as they get older.

Of course, doing the Feingold Diet is not your gateway to health, but it is definitely a start and a baby step in the right direction. Most families are not willing to go from eating the typical American diet to eating all whole foods and nothing processed. Feingold helps you make wiser choices and makes you think about what's going into the foods you are feeding your family. From there, it's in your hands.

What If I Don't Have the Money?

I know this is a real issue for so many people. You might be convinced that the diet is worth the money, but you don't have the actual money to spend on a membership or even the food. What do you do then? Whenever I face an obstacle in life, I go to two places: God, and the Internet!

When we first started Feingold, I had some reservations about how we were going to afford the more expensive food as I was not a good cook. I prayed and trusted that if God wanted us to do this diet he was going to provide the money to pay for it. We have been blessed and although our grocery bills are higher, we have never had a problem paying our bills. As I've discussed though, some of it was just a trade-off as to where we were spending our money.

After praying, next I have to do research. Researching and educating yourself is not going to pay for your groceries, but you can learn ways to save money and be more cost efficient so you can stretch your dollar farther.

I joined www.moneysavingmom.com. This is currently a free resource. You can sign up to receive e-mail alerts for coupons and sales at the stores that you shop at. I have scored some really good deals from Whole Foods and other stores like Target. Read my post on All Natural Couponing (see the References section for link) for more details. [1]

Couponing is not a get rich quick (or get lots of free products quick) scheme. It's a slow and steady wins the race. Every once in a while I find some really good deals and I stock up. It takes time to learn the ropes and coupon well, but if I was low on cash, I would definitely spend more time couponing.

Check out books on saving money on groceries. Steve and Annette Economides are the authors of the "America's Cheapest Family" books.[2] I have two of them listed in the resource section at the end of this book. They have some great tips on how to live frugally and save money on groceries. I was excited to learn that I had already incorporated many of their suggestions.

Feingold members also suggest trying the "Caveman" diet, which is similar to the Paleo Diet. Feingold has a link which explains this, currently at http://feingold.org/caveman.html. [3] You are basically eating how cavemen used to. Think meats, fruits, rice, veggies, nuts, and eggs.

If you cannot afford the Feingold program, you can apply for financial assistance from Feingold. E-mail them at help@feingold.org to inquire about it. Currently, the discount for those eligible is about half off, after providing proper documentation showing your need.

Do your best to read labels (see chapter 10) and continue to educate yourself on food ingredients. Check out my list of resources at the end of this book for good web sites, books, and documentaries. Join the Feingold Association of the United States Facebook group. Search Pinterest for Feingold recipes.

Cook and stick to the basics. Think whole, real food such as fruits, vegetables, homemade soups, muffins, pancakes, and homemade desserts. When you bake, freeze your leftovers. Avoid as many processed foods as possible unless you know they are clean.

I also wrote a post entitled, "3-Day Trial of the Feingold Diet."[4] Some people have stretched this for two weeks. While ingredients and approved foods can change at any time, this 3-day guide might be helpful and give you an idea of the kinds of things your child can eat on stage one of the diet. Another helpful post I wrote is entitled, "Not Quite Ready to Start the Feingold Diet? 30 Simple Changes Anyone Can Make."

And what if you can afford the membership but not the food? This is a common problem. You're not alone. Many people are doing the diet on a strict budget. It is possible. You will have to cook more. There's no way around that if you want to save money. If you don't have the time to cook because you work or have young kids, let me just say that there may be more hours in your day than you think.

I've read some really good books on time management. "*168 Hours, You Have More Time Than You Think*" by Laura Vanderkam is a good one.[5] She suggests keeping track of your time for one full week, down to the minutes. Where are you currently spending your time? This is kind of like when you do a budget and keep track of where all your money is going. If you are not conscious of how you spend your time, it tends to slip away from you idly.

I think it also has to do with where your priorities are. You might have to rearrange some things for a while until you get the diet underway and established. If you watch TV or go on social media a lot, consider cutting back. Those two things seem to take up a lot more time than we realize.

Don't think that you have to do it all at once. Take just one or two days and commit it to baking, cooking, and/or researching recipes. I know of one working mom who cooks and bakes every Sunday for the following week. When you have nothing stocked in your freezer, of course in the beginning it seems daunting. But slowly, you'll get it fully stocked and then you'll just be replenishing one item at a time instead of starting from scratch on everything.

I might make muffins one day and a couple days later, some pancakes. Those will last a couple weeks and some things last a couple months. If I had nothing in my freezer, I'd have to make pancakes, muffins, cupcakes, spaghetti sauce, chicken nuggets, French toast, soup, chili, chicken stew, etc. all at once to stock it. I certainly didn't make all of those in one day or in one month even. It takes time to stock your freezer when you are first starting out. It won't happen in one day so try not to feel overwhelmed like you have to do everything all at once. That won't happen and you'll get burned out if you try.

And if you don't know how to freeze leftovers, here's a quick run-down. For things like muffins or cupcakes with frosting, put them on a plate in your freezer for about an hour. Just long enough till the frosting is set and hard. Then transfer them to a large sealable plastic freezer bag. Make sure you label them with the date and contents. Very important!

For things like pancakes, French toast, or chicken nuggets, I usually just let them cool completely then lay them flat in the plastic bag. They can overlap slightly but not too much or they'll stick together when you try to take them out later. Or you can also freeze these on a plate first too.

For soups and sauces, just let them cool. Sometimes I put them in the fridge first. Then transfer to plastic freezer bags. I use quart size for soups and do about two cups for one serving size. Don't stack soups in the freezer on top of each other before they have frozen or they will get stuck together. And that's pretty much it.

You'll also have to remember to take some things out the night before to thaw. I've broken more than one jar using hot water trying to thaw them out. For muffins, I warm them up in our toaster oven, and for cupcakes, just allow an hour or so to thaw, or eat them cold! My kids like to.

Above all else, don't give up! Just because you can't afford the program or all of the food doesn't mean you can't make changes for the better. *Any* amount of change you can make for your family is better than nothing. Although I will add here that if you are dealing with a child with definite ADHD, doing the Feingold program 100% is really the only way you are going to see the results you are looking for. But, don't let that deter you from making the changes that you can today.

Chapter 9

Is It Difficult?

When asking if this diet is difficult or hard, one first has to answer the question, what does hard mean to you? For me hard was the stress of dealing with an extremely hyper child day in and day out. There were no pleasant trips to the mall or store for us. It was get in and get out as quickly as possible.

Hard is feeling like you are to blame for your child's misbehavior. Hard is not being able to get together with friends because you know that your child cannot control himself enough. Hard is seeing the remorse in your child's eyes after they have misbehaved and sensing that they couldn't help it and didn't want to misbehave. Hard is the stress of going to parent teacher conferences, knowing you are going to hear a bad report. Hard is when you get calls from your child's teacher threatening to kick your child out of class. Hard is watching your child's self-esteem plummet. Hard is having to constantly discipline your child. Hard is watching your child struggle to concentrate and do their homework. Hard is listening to all the unwanted ill advice of family and friends. Hard is when your spouse is unsupportive and you feel alone in your struggles. Hard is wanting to see your child succeed in life, and not knowing how to help them.

Add your own things to the list. Some people have had their child kicked out of more than one school or daycare. Some parents have reluctantly put their kids on ADHD medication, only to agonize over the side effects, not knowing what other choices they had, and trying to do what was best for their child.

If you ask those of us who are dealing with an ADHD child if a change in diet is hard, you're going to get this answer: "It is nowhere *near* as hard as dealing with my child when they are not on the diet. Not even close." Is it hard at first to make all these changes and find new foods and recipes? Yes, but it gets much easier as time goes on, and it is SO worth it.

Once you start seeing results, the thought of it being hard starts to dissipate. For us, the benefits far outweighed the inconveniences. If you start to think that it's not worth all the extra effort, just let your child eat off diet once. You will quickly regain your motivation and be reminded of why you do this diet.

Is it a lifestyle adjustment? Yes, in a good way. Social functions will require more planning and to some, it will feel like a big inconvenience. However, for me personally, it was still an improvement. We could now go to more social functions and actually enjoy ourselves and feel less stressed because my son was under control. We didn't have to leave early or skip the function because of my son's behavior. It really didn't feel like a huge inconvenience to us once we got used to it. It felt like a huge blessing!

A seasoned Feingold member compared starting the diet to having your first baby. That first month with your new baby, you are completely overwhelmed. But soon, through trial and error, the right baby products, and a little help from others, you learn all there is to know about caring for your baby. By that second or third baby, it seems like a piece of cake and you really enjoy the experience because now you know what you're doing and it just becomes second nature.

For those who do not have a child with some of these issues, you might be wondering if you want to make this kind of investment with your time and money. What *is* so hard about the diet?

Finding the Food

At first it can be hard to find all these new foods. You'll look through the Feingold shopping guide and see some foods that you may not be familiar with, and then have to try to hunt them down. You may not know which store you can find them at. This was the part I hated the most. Don't worry, this problem is only temporary. Once you figure out what store the item you want is in, you're fine.

I remember searching for California Baby shampoo for my toddler. It was listed in the shopping guide, but I had no idea where I was going to find it. I searched several different stores. I finally went on the Feingold message board and found out I could find it at Whole Foods or possibly my local health food store. My local health food store? Never been there. I never would have figured out that I would need to look there had I not asked. You can also find this shampoo online and in some Target stores.

This is one of the reasons why I listed out my shopping list by store on my web site. [1] That was my biggest hurdle starting the diet – not knowing which store I could find these items at. With two young kids, I didn't have time to search each store for each item. Feingold also has a few shopping lists by store on their web site and in the files section of their Facebook group for reference.

I then went on to figure out which store sold the product for the cheapest price. The prices could vary substantially from store to store. We have a Woodman's store near us, and they sell a lot of the same foods as Whole Foods for a lot less.

You will also probably have to shop at new stores if you are used to only shopping at your local grocery store. Before Feingold, I never shopped at Whole Foods, Trader Joe's, or my local health food store. Now I shop at about five different stores (keep in mind we are also GFCF and a family with four kids). I try to hit one of these stores once a week so that I'm doing one of these about once a month, sometimes more. Then I occasionally go to my local grocery store (Meijer) and Wal-Mart or Target.

It's not that I can't find Feingold approved items at regular grocery stores, it's just that I can go to these other stores (Woodman's especially) and find more of what I need in one place, and at a cheaper price. I also shop at Sam's Club and Costco as needed.

Bringing Your Own Food

Before heading out somewhere, it takes me twice as long to get ready because I am packing food. This doesn't bother me because it is a minor inconvenience compared to dealing with my kids' behavior afterwards for the next two days if I don't. If we are not going to be gone long, I just prefer to feed my kids before we head out the door and just bring along snacks and dessert.

I try to pack as much as I can the night before heading out for a day, so that there is less to do in the morning. Fruit and other sides and snacks get cut up and ready the night before. In the morning it's usually a matter of boiling a few hot dogs and throwing them in a thermos, and making a couple of sandwiches. Sometimes I'll bring a microwavable meal along (like an Ian's chicken nugget meal or an individual Annie's macaroni and cheese packet), depending on where we are going.

You do have the option of picking up Feingold approved fast food, and we have done that many times. I always bring along at least a dessert if we are going to a party though. If we are going to a theme park, the zoo, or the water park for the day, then I pack all our food in a cooler. I'm saving money and we're eating healthier, so for me, it's not a big deal.

For some people, this is going to be a big adjustment. Having the right "supplies" is very helpful. I have a nice cooler back pack that I got online from Target. For ideas on what to pack, you can visit my web site. It largely depends on what your kids like.

I have a couple of really nice food thermoses that I got on Amazon by Nissan Thermos. Forget the character ones at Target. Cute, yes, but I've found that they only keep the food hot for about two to three hours. It works OK if your child has an early lunch, but I've found the Nissan ones work much better, especially if you have a long day ahead of you. I also have a bigger Nissan thermal thermos as well that keeps juice or water cold for twenty-four hours.

We have cupcake holders from www.cupacake.com. These will hold a frosted cupcake or muffin upright and keep it from being tossed around and the frosting getting destroyed - perfect for class parties or birthday parties. I also use them to pack muffins in for lunch. Small Tupperware containers work well too but if you have a frosted cupcake, the Cup-A-Cake containers are really nice. My only complaint is they don't hold larger cupcakes or muffins very well. I'm hoping they increase the size of their holders soon.

If you only have to pack for one or two children, be thankful. I'm packing food for four kids and one adult when we go out places. If I was Michelle Duggar from the reality TV show, "19 Kids and Counting", and had nineteen kids, I think I'd be in trouble. Always something to be thankful for!

And what if you are going to a theme park or water park that doesn't allow you to bring food in? Well, all I have to say is, I've never been turned away once. You may have to give them your best Mama Bear look though. I've always taken food in. I just tell them my kids have allergies and can't eat any of the food in there.

If they want to get all technical, tell them you are protected under the Americans With Disabilities Act. If they ask to see a doctor's note, tell them it is illegal for them to ask for that according to HIPPA laws. They should stop there and let you right in. If not, they don't know the laws. Ask for a manager.

If you want to play it safe, you can also call or e-mail the place you are going ahead of time and tell them your situation. They may give you an e-mail approval ahead of time that you can show to the security personnel. Some people also just leave a cooler in their car and go out to their car for lunch. We've done that for lunch, but with younger kids, this doesn't always work. I have a child who eats every two hours so going out to the car every time she is hungry isn't feasible.

Cooking More

Do you have to cook more? Yes. The Feingold Association likes to say that you don't have to, but when it comes down to it, you will be cooking more. How much more is up to you. You can buy all prepackaged foods, but if you're interested in healthier eating, do you really want to? Plus, it can get expensive. Do we use prepackaged foods sometimes? Absolutely, but I still cook and bake too.

Cooking is something you can ease in to. You don't have to do it all at once. I didn't. I had to figure out which kitchen supplies I was going to need. I did not have a stand-alone mixer - never had a need for one. Once I acquired all these kitchen items, I understood why my mom was such a good cook. It was all about using the right tools.

With my mom being such a good cook, you would think it would have rubbed off on me. Nope. She was a good cook. Why did I need to cook? Even when I first got married, she would have us over for dinner at least once a week.

Then, something happened. My parents got a winter home in Florida. Panic set in. My mom would no longer be stocking my freezer with homemade spaghetti sauce, homemade pizzas, chili, lasagna, and cookies. After a serious food drought of a couple of months, I decided I was going to have to learn how to cook.

I've learned some things over the years. I discovered my cookies never turned out right because I was using a cheap dark pan. I had no idea. I got a nice silver air bake pan from Bed Bath & Beyond that cooked evenly and I never again had a problem with crunchy cookies. I also used a cookie scooper so the cookies all came out the same size, and cooked evenly. No more having some cookies done before others.

I learned how to cut onions so my eyes didn't water like crazy. I had never cut an onion before. I throw them in the freezer now for about ten minutes before cutting them, and then run them under cold water while I'm peeling the skin, and then breathe through my nose instead of my mouth. Problem solved (usually).

I learned that a garlic clove is not the same as a whole head of garlic (good to know), and that you have to peel it and what minced means (chop it up into tiny pieces). I learned most of this by way of phone calls to my mom or Internet searches. You can find anything you want to know about cooking online. You can usually find a YouTube video on it too.

I learned that when you cook a rotisserie chicken, the legs need to be on top. The first time I cooked one, I placed it in the pan upside down. When I went to cut it, I couldn't figure out why there was hardly any meat on this thing. I found a lot of the good meat was on the bottom. I told my mom about it and figured out I put the bird in upside down. Lesson learned.

Are you getting the picture? If you can't cook, don't worry. You can learn. I don't think anyone could have been any worse than I was when we started the diet. It wasn't that I was a moron or incompetent. I just never found the need to cook. We were happy eating out of a can or box, or eating out. If you already cook, you are way ahead of the game. Now all you need to do is make sure you are cooking with the right ingredients.

Worried that you're going to have to spend a lot of money on new kitchen supplies? I didn't get everything at once. My mom had some things that she gave me. The rest I just asked for for my birthday,

Christmas, Mother's Day, or I used those holidays as excuses to buy them for myself. Then, over time, I ended up with everything I have now. You can improvise. The only thing I would say was really helpful was a nice baking sheet for cookies. The rest are conveniences.

Putting It All In Perspective

If you ask me if Feingold is difficult, I would say it *is* in the beginning because you have a lot to learn, read, and cook, and that takes time. Meanwhile your family has to eat. It's a big adjustment at first. It gets so much easier though. Once you have these things down, you just go into repeat mode.

Once you know your son likes a certain cereal, you continue to buy it. Once you find a recipe your family likes, you make it. You won't be trying and experimenting with foods forever. It's only in the beginning, and then after that, you can slowly add to or adjust your grocery list and meals as needed.

Of course, there will be times even when you've been on the diet for a while, when you feel overwhelmed. You may wish your kids could just eat what everyone else's kids are eating. I remember feeling that way. I had two little ones and a new baby to take care of and I was just falling into that complaining mode. In those times, I find it helpful to have a change in perspective.

There are other families who have much more to deal with. They may be dealing with cancer or some other disease. There are families who have life threatening food allergies. There are families who are struggling just to even feed their families due to finances.

I met a woman at a birthday party whose child had a condition where she had to puree all of his food and feed him through a tube that was inserted through an opening in his stomach. I will no longer complain about having to make my daughter her own cupcake to bring along to parties! At least she can eat a cupcake. If this child went to a birthday party, he couldn't eat anything.

For me, with four kids, I can get stressed about having to feed so many kids. Then I turn on TLC and watch *19 Kids and Counting.* Yikes! I can't even imagine trying to feed nineteen kids every day, three meals a day, and snacks. Then I always feel better about *only* having four kids to feed and I'm thankful instead of complaining about it.

You can watch the show and think that Michelle Duggar has a lot of help with the older kids, and that's true. However, if you read her first book, *The Duggars!: 20 and Counting,* [2] she explains that she had to do it all herself for a long time while her kids were still young. It's a really good book. I highly recommend it because it will make you rethink your entire role as a mother and it may help when you are feeling overwhelmed by a change in diet and lifestyle.

When Hard Becomes Even Harder

Four years after we started Feingold, I was feeling really good about cooking and the fact that I had a good handle on the diet. I loved cooking and I loved food! Instead of the McDonald's queen, I was Martha Stewart. I felt like I could make anything my kids wanted. I had my personal cookbook (a binder with all of my favorite recipes printed and in sheet protectors), and was baking pretty much every weekend with the kids just because it was fun. Life was good.

Then, life hit the fan. My 12-month-old son had a grand mal febrile seizure and almost died in my arms. Four months later, he had another grand mal seizure. I remembered watching Jenny McCarthy on Oprah talking about doing the GFCF diet for her son who had seizures. I immediately went out and bought Jenny McCarthy's book and read it in one night. The next day, I started the GFCF diet cold turkey for my son and for my daughter as well, whom I suspected had autism.

Suddenly, my life was turned upside down and all my recipes were useless. I had to start over. Just when I had everything figured out, God threw in a monkey wrench. It was time to find new recipes, learn and read a whole lot more about nutrition, seizures, autism, biomed, and supplements.

I had my kids tested for allergies and had to remove even more foods. Now, I think back and wish we could *just* do Feingold. What a treat that would be, and when I compare Feingold to doing GFCF plus, it seems like a piece of cake! It didn't seem like it at the time. When I started the diet, it *was* difficult, but now I see how much more difficult it could have been.

I'm very thankful that God allowed us to transition slowly into a GFCF diet. I already knew how to cook and we were already used to bringing our own food places. It wasn't as hard as it could have been, had we needed to go straight to Feingold plus gluten free, dairy free, egg free, peanut free, soy free, low oxalate, and more.

At least with the Feingold Diet, you are not eliminating whole food groups. If your child wants ice cream, they can have ice cream. It's just going to be a different brand than they were eating before.

Philippians 2:14 says, "Do everything without complaining or arguing." I've learned my lesson on that one. I know it could be a lot worse. I'm just thankful that my children have the ability to eat. I will never again (hopefully) let myself grumble and complain about a diet that my child needs.

We have moved way beyond Feingold now, but we still do the Feingold Diet as a base to all of our other diets. Even though we are GFCF, we certainly don't eat artificials or preservatives. Feingold will always be a part of our lifestyle.

As for doing things that stretch beyond the Feingold Diet like other special diets, supplements, and biomed, I will address that in another book. That's a huge topic. Feingold isn't necessarily about eating as nutritiously as possible, although that should be the goal of every parent.

As with anything, you need to use common sense. Just because ice cream and candy are approved doesn't mean you are going to feed that to your child every day. The Feingold Diet allows you to set your own limits on how much sugar you allow your child to eat, or what questionable additives you want to include in your family's diet or not.

Chapter 10

How Do I Read Labels?

The truth is it's hard to read labels! Anyone trying to do the Feingold Diet on their own can attest to this. Going into a grocery store and trying to tell if an item has any harmful chemicals in it is mind boggling. You will likely spend a couple of hours in the store and still end up with a cart full of artificial-laden food despite all your best efforts.

There are some things that you can watch out for though. Over time, you will get better at recognizing what is and is not truly natural, despite any claims on the packaging. While it's best to rely on Feingold's information, below is some information that will help you understand and read labels a little better. If you see certain ingredients listed on a label, you will know automatically that the product is not an acceptable food.

Ingredients You Want to Avoid

There are three groups of additives that you want to avoid completely on the Feingold Diet. Those are artificial colors (dyes), artificial flavors, and the preservatives BHT, TBHQ, and BHA. These three groups are avoided on both stage one and stage two of the diet.

Artificial Colors

These are things like red dye (sometimes with a number after it like red #40 or yellow FD&C #6, blue #1, etc.) Sometimes the dyes and numbers are preceded by FD&C. FD&C stands for Food, Drug, and Cosmetics. Yellow dye can also be listed as tartrazine.[1] Artificial colors may be listed simply as "colors added". If not listed as natural colors, it is much more likely to be artificial.

Caramel color is one that is sometimes natural and sometimes artificial. Natural caramel color is made by melting sugar. The artificial caramel color is made by combining sugars with ammonia and sulfites under high pressure and high temperatures. This causes a carcinogenic end product. [2]

I have found that when caramel color is listed in a more "natural" product, it is often an approved product. If listed in a mainstream product, it is more likely to be artificial.

Artificial Flavors

Sometimes manufacturers will just list an ingredient as "flavors." Those are usually artificial. If the product is truly natural, you would think they would take advantage of that fact and list it as such. But, even if it does say natural flavors, it could still contain harmful additives, so "natural flavors" will always be a questionable ingredient and one I rely on Feingold for.

Vanillin is an artificial flavor used in a lot of chocolate and vanilla flavored products.[3] Vanillin is also used in some cheap imitation vanilla extracts. If a product contains vanilla (like cookies, or baked goods), they may not list out the ingredients that make up the vanilla, which may include vanillin. If a product lists vanillin or vanilla flavors, it is usually the synthetic form and you will want to avoid that product. When a product lists vanilla extract, there is more chance that it is in the natural form.

So, to recap, if a product lists vanillin, you want to avoid it. If a product lists vanilla flavors, it is probably artificial and you will want to avoid it, unless it is Feingold approved. If a product lists vanilla, it is questionable, and you will want to verify with Feingold. If a product lists vanilla extract, it is probably OK, but best to verify with Feingold. See why it's hard to read labels?

Natural Flavors and Natural Colors

Watch out for natural flavors and natural colors. These may or may not be truly natural. Companies are not required to list all the ingredients within their flavorings. Something with natural flavors could contain twenty to thirty different chemicals in it, some of which may contain artificial ingredients. [4] They often hide MSG under the name "natural flavors."

BHA and BHT are often hidden in annatto and beta-carotene, which are found in many cheeses and margarines to preserve the orange or yellow color. The preservatives help prevent rancidity and help the products retain the color longer. They may simply list the annatto and beta-carotene as "natural colors." Annatto and beta-carotene themselves are acceptable ingredients. Annatto comes from the seeds of a tropical plant. [5] Some people experience allergic reactions such as hives from annatto, even though it is from a natural source. So, just be mindful of that. Beta-carotene is found in vegetables and fruits like carrots and tomatoes. [6]

Annatto and beta-carotene become unacceptable when they have preservatives added to them. The preservatives may or may not be listed on the ingredient label. Often, you will see vitamin A palmitate listed as an ingredient in cheese products which contain annatto, and the preservatives may be included in the vitamin A palmitate. See below.

Preservatives – BHT, TBHQ, and BHA

Some preservatives are acceptable on the Feingold Diet and some are not. BHT (Butylated Hydroxytoluene), TBHQ (Tertiary Butylhydroquinone), and BHA (Butylated Hydroxyanisole), are not accepted. If you see any of these listed in the ingredients, avoid that product. These preservatives may be listed as simply "antioxidants."

Manufacturers are not required by law to list things they use in the packaging. BHT and BHA are commonly used in cereal packaging and in juice or milk cartons. [7] These preservatives absorb right into the food or drink.

These preservatives are also used a lot in oils and sprays. If a bakery sprays a pan with oil containing BHT, they aren't going to list that on the ingredients of the finished baked good or bread, but BHT is certainly getting into the food.

Most fast food companies use oil containing one of these three preservatives, which is why very few restaurant fries are approved. The same is true of pizza restaurants. They often spray the pans with oils containing BHT, TBHQ, or BHA.

Other preservatives you want to avoid are artificial sweeteners like Aspartame (NutraSweet, Equal), Sucralose (Splenda), and Saccharine

(Sweet N'Low). These are found in a lot of diet drinks, low calorie foods, gum, and yogurts.

Vitamin A Palmitate

Vitamin A Palmitate can have BHT added to preserve it. This will not always be listed in the ingredients. Vitamin A Palmitate is often found in milk. If you see vitamin A Palmitate listed, you will have to contact the manufacturer to try to find out if the product contains preservatives. My friend called one manufacturer of an organic rice milk which had vitamin A palmitate in it. She found out that they did in fact add BHT, which was not listed on the ingredients. Sadly, even organic products are not immune to using preservatives and chemicals.

Optional Additives To Avoid

The additives listed below are ones that our family tries to avoid for health reasons. Feingold includes them as acceptable on the diet. However, they do let people know that they are in a product for those who wish to avoid them. In the shopping guide, a food that contains corn syrup and MSG would have these letters listed after the product name: (CS, MSG).

MSG

MSG stands for monosodium glutamate. We avoid it. It gives my son headaches. MSG is a flavor enhancer among other things. Many fast food and sit down restaurants add MSG to their foods.

Have you ever craved fast food and then as you are eating, you think to yourself, "This doesn't even taste that good. Why did I want this so bad and why am I still eating it?" That's thanks to MSG. It tricks the brain into thinking that the food tastes better than it actually does. It is addicting and makes you want to eat more of the food. When they feed MSG to rats, they get fat. Google the phrase, "MSG makes you fat" and you will find several interesting articles. [8]

MSG is also an excitotoxin. [9] Just the name excitotoxin makes me not want to give it to my kids. MSG also kills brain cells. I tell my kids that MSG puts holes in their brain, because it actually does. They talk about this in the documentary, *Sweet Misery*. This documentary also covers the dangers of aspartame found in many diet drinks and other foods. (Aspartame is not acceptable on the Feingold Diet, but MSG is. More on why later.)

They often hide MSG under different ingredient names. [9] MSG can be concealed under the names autolyzed yeast, hydrolyzed vegetable protein (HPV), natural flavors, bouillon, natural chicken flavoring, broth, and many more. If MSG was not harmful, then why would they try to hide it? As it is, food manufacturers go to great lengths to conceal it.

My brother thinks it is so funny that my kids know all about MSG and know what it stands for. Laugh all you want. At least my kids don't have holes in their heads. One day when my son was eating some chicken that I made that he wasn't too fond of, he asked, "Can you add some MSG to this?" Smarty pants.

There are also two good books that have been written about MSG. They are *MSG: The Slow Poisoning of America* by John Erb [10], and *Excitotoxins: The Taste That Kills* by Dr. Russell Blaylock [11]. The titles alone scare me.

MSG is one of the few things that Feingold leaves up to the member to decide if they want to avoid or not. Part of that reason is because of how difficult it is to track MSG in products. It can be hidden in so many ingredients that it would be difficult to be certain if a product does contain MSG or not. They do however educate members on the dangers of MSG in the Feingold e-newsletters. I knew nothing about MSG before we started Feingold. In reading and talking to other Feingold members, I've learned MSG is not something I want anywhere near myself or my kids on a regular basis. I'm thankful that Feingold inquires about the presence of MSG in products, and when a company admits to its presence, Feingold lists it out for those of us who want to avoid it. Thankfully, it isn't in too many of the Feingold accepted foods.

Nitrates & Nitrites

Nitrates and nitrites (abbreviated as N in the shopping guide) are often added to processed deli meats, ham, bacon, hot dogs, and a few other foods as a preservative or color enhancer. We avoid them because they tend to give people headaches, and my kids and I are prone to headaches. Nitrites can occur naturally in foods too, as in the case of some vegetables. However, some studies have shown the synthetic forms are carcinogenic (*The China Study* [12] book also states this), so I would rather just avoid them.

Sodium Benzoate

Sodium benzoate is another preservative that is acceptable on Feingold, but some choose to avoid it. We do. Sodium benzoate (abbreviated as SB in the shopping guide) gives my son and I a headache, while for some kids, it makes them go wild. Sodium benzoate is found in many sodas including Sprite (Sprite is considered Feingold acceptable in the fast food guide).

My kids went on vacation with another family member last summer and the joke about my son when they got back was, "Don't give him Sprite!" It was like a Gremlin to water. They learned quickly that my six-year-old went wild from Sprite. It was likely from the sodium benzoate as he can have corn syrup and sugar on occasion and not go completely wild. We usually stick to Sierra Mist if I let him have pop. (Sierra Mist is one that is not officially approved, but many members use it without a problem.)

Natural News posted an article entitled, *Sodium Benzoate Is a Preservative That Promotes Cancer and Kills Healthy Cells.* [13] No wonder it gives me a headache. Sodium benzoate is the cheapest mold inhibitor on the market. Benzoic acid is found in low levels in some foods, but sodium benzoate is made in a lab by reacting sodium hydroxide with benzoic acid. Sounds like a chemistry experiment! The FDA claims it is safe in low levels, but don't ever combine it with vitamin C or E, as benzene will form. Remember that! Or just avoid it! Benzene is a known carcinogen. [13]

Corn Syrup is Evil, and Other Names for It

As I mentioned in an earlier chapter, we were on the Feingold Diet for six months before I realized that corn syrup was a problem for my son. One of the first things I want to ask if anyone says that the diet isn't working as well as they had hoped is, "Have you taken out corn syrup?"

Corn syrup is one of the things I think Feingold should add to their list of unacceptable ingredients. The stuff is nasty. Watch the documentary

King Corn [14]. They show how corn syrup is made. They also share some pretty eye-opening things about cows in America and how they are fed. We switched to grass fed beef after watching this movie.

Feingold does list out corn syrup (CS) though for those who want to avoid it, which I am incredibly thankful for. Like other harmful additives, it is often hidden under other names. Some common names for corn syrup are dextrose, fructose, maltodextrin, of course the infamous high-fructose corn syrup (HFCS), and the newest is corn sugar. I call it pure evil.

Corn producers are concerned that high fructose corn syrup is getting a bad rap (as it should). How many products do you see now that say "No High-Fructose Corn Syrup"? But here's the kicker: many of those still contain regular corn syrup, which in my opinion is just high fructose syrup with a little less kick. Corn syrup is corn syrup, no matter what you call it.

Studies have also come out showing that almost half of the products they tested containing high-fructose corn syrup, also contained traces of mercury. [15] That doesn't surprise me based on the reactions we see with corn syrup. No amount of mercury is safe. It's difficult to know which products containing high-fructose corn syrup also contain mercury. Your best bet is to stay away from all of it. HFCS is most commonly found in sodas and fast food, but it is found in many foods.

How Corn Syrup Affects Our Family

How did I realize corn syrup was a problem for my son? When we started the Feingold Diet I immediately noticed that my son was calmer. However, I noticed that he was suddenly overly emotional and crying over things that he normally would not get upset about. Instead of being hyper, sometimes he was angry, weepy, and aggressive. He would be playing his video games and if he lost, he would yell at the TV and cry. This wasn't like him.

At preschool, the teacher pulled me aside one day and asked if everything was okay at home because of the way he was acting at school. He was suddenly becoming upset and emotional on the playground. He was normally a very happy kid. I even questioned whether this new behavior I was seeing was better than the pre-Feingold one, but I didn't give up.

It took a few months, but I discovered that he could not tolerate corn syrup, which he was eating frequently. I don't think I ever noticed this before because he was eating dyes at the same time as corn syrup. The extreme hyperactivity probably masked the behaviors that corn syrup was causing. I would rather be around my kids when they are hyper and out of control from dyes, than angry, aggressive, and crying from corn syrup, but we avoid both now obviously.

On the Feingold message board, I found that corn syrup causes the same reaction in many adults. I stay away from corn syrup myself because corn syrup makes me angry too. I also figured out that he did not do well with chocolate either. Chocolate caused some of the same reactions as corn syrup.

Once we removed corn syrup and chocolate, he was much better. In talking with other moms, it seems that some kids with zinc deficiencies (which many ADHD kids have) often show behavioral problems from eating chocolate. Chocolate is a food that affects mood. Dark chocolate is high in zinc and magnesium. If kids are low in zinc or magnesium, they may crave chocolate. [16]

It is commonly known in the biomed community of parents, that when you first start to supplement with a vitamin a child is deficient in, they may react to it at first while their body adjusts. It usually takes at least three weeks for the body to get acclimated. Sometimes when you correct this vitamin deficiency, the kids are better able to handle chocolate. My kids do handle chocolate better today, but we also supplement with calcium, magnesium, and zinc daily.

And as much as I don't like corn syrup, my kids do eat it on occasion if we eat out - the same with MSG. We try our best to avoid it, but it doesn't *always* happen. There are some times when you just have to choose the lesser of two evils. If we have to eat out, I'd rather choose something with MSG and corn syrup, then something with MSG, corn syrup, red dyes, and artificial flavors. Not everything in the Feingold shopping guide has corn syrup and MSG. Much of it does not.

GMO's

GMO's (Genetically Modified Organisms) are genetically engineered plants or animals.   They are foods that have been developed through the experimental combination of genes from different species. GMO's cannot be found in nature. Most GMO seeds were made to withstand the application of harmful herbicides and pesticides in order to make the plants more insect and disease resistant, and to yield bigger harvests. [17]

GMO's were first introduced into our food supply in the 1970's. Many other countries ban the use of GMO's or greatly reduce their use. There are no long term studies on the effects of eating GMO's. [17] We simply do not know what eating GMO foods daily for a long period of time can do to our bodies. Our kids may be the guinea pigs. There's a documentary called, *Genetic Roulette* that discusses GMO's. [18]

If you buy 100% organic, you have a better chance of avoiding GMO's (although some regulations may change that in the future). Some companies state, "Contains No GMO's" right on their packaging. The subject of GMO's is a big one.

We try to avoid GMO's when we can. Some of the biggest GMO crops are currently corn, canola, soy, sugar beets, and a few more. Also at risk are meat products – beef, milk, cheese, eggs, and the like because the animals are being fed GMO corn and soy products. [17] Two states currently require GMO labeling on products, while many others are considering legislation on it. And as of 2018, Whole Foods ® plans to label GMO products. [19]

If I am buying a corn product, I try to buy organic. I use organic corn starch and organic corn meal when baking. If I'm buying a product with corn or soy in it, I can pretty much expect that it's going to contain GMO's unless I buy organic. Unfortunately, corn and soy are in so many products, it makes it hard to avoid GMO's. They estimate that at least 80 percent of processed foods contain GMO's.[17] Even more reason to cook your food from scratch and try to avoid processed foods.

Where and when we can buy organic, we do. GMO's are accepted on the Feingold Diet but some people choose to avoid them as there is concern over the safety of ingesting genetically modified foods. Feingold does not list out which foods contain GMO's. Why not? Partly because GMO's are not currently researched by most manufacturers. And partly because so many processed foods contain GMO's. Sometimes I feel like if I want to avoid GMO's, I'm going to have to stick to foods from my backyard garden. Thankfully, this is getting better through education of the public and the demands we are putting on manufacturers to use better ingredients.

As stated earlier, the Feingold Diet is not about eating the healthiest foods possible, though that should be the goal. It's a diet which has been shown to help ADHD and other symptoms by avoiding specific artificial ingredients and salicylates. The food guide lists out which processed foods do not contain these particularly harmful chemicals.

Would kids experience even more improvement by avoiding GMO's? Probably. But, it would also mean narrowing down your choices drastically. For many people, it would make doing the diet nearly impossible. As well, many, many families have experienced life-changing results just by following the Feingold Diet as is. Avoiding GMO's is something that some families look into after they've learned and established the Feingold Diet. If you want to learn more about GMO's and how to avoid them, I would suggest following Vani Hari, aka "Food Babe" at www.foodbabe.com, and also follow her Facebook page.

Help! I'm Overwhelmed!

I included information about the above additives, not to overwhelm, but as information to tuck in the back of your head. You do not have to eliminate these things right away, but in the interest of better health, it's something you might want to look into in the future. But if you're new to all of this, just start with the basic Feingold Diet first. My only recommendation is to try to avoid corn syrup as well.

Why does Feingold include corn syrup, MSG, and other not so healthy additives as acceptable foods on the diet? Well, on a similar note, someone asked Dr. Feingold why he included sugar on the diet. His answer was, "I bit off a little more than I could handle with the salicylate business." [20] He was already causing a stir by telling people to pull dyes, artificial flavors, preservatives and salicylates. I think a lot of people wouldn't even consider the diet if they had to avoid sugar too. And, Dr. Feingold found that when people avoided just those things eliminated in the Feingold Diet, they saw results.

It's kind of the same concept. Is sugar a problem for most kids? Yes. Feingold leaves it up to the parents to use good judgment and common sense, and not overdo it just because sugar is approved on the diet. I believe when Dr. Feingold started this diet back in the 1970's, they weren't using as much of these other harmful additives (like MSG, corn syrup, and the like). There weren't as many studies done yet on the dangers of these newer additives. Now there are. If Feingold moved corn syrup to the unaccepted category, many foods would have to be removed from the shopping guide. As well, there are some kids who do not react to corn syrup. Some of those parents allow their kids to have corn syrup on occasion. It's really a personal decision.

Is There Any Truth in Labeling?

As stated already, the problem is manufacturers do not have to list every single ingredient. If a food contains less than .5 grams per serving of an ingredient, they are not required by law to list it. [21]

No matter how well you can read labels, you still may end up with a product with harmful chemicals in it. Food manufacturers also may be using ingredients that were produced by an outside supplier. For example, a chocolate chip cookie mix might list chocolate chips which they acquired from an outside supplier. They may not list out the ingredients in those chocolate chips which may contain vanillin, an artificial flavor. They may even state that their product is all natural and contains no added artificial flavors. The producer of the chocolate chip cookie mix did not add the artificial flavors, but their chocolate chip supplier may have.

So how does Feingold know what is acceptable? They contact the companies in writing using a form and ask very specific questions. They also require information from all of the manufacturer's suppliers. I'm very thankful that I don't have to spend hours at the store reading labels! I can open the Feingold shopping guide and see a list of foods that are acceptable and free of dyes and other harmful additives.

Feingold helps you make better choices with the processed foods that are out there. As a parent, you have to take it from there and take ownership and responsibility for your family's health. Once I learned and mastered the Feingold Diet, I continued to learn about food and health, and continued to make changes for the better. We choose to reduce the amount of processed foods in our diet and choose to eat out less often. We eat more organic foods then we did before starting the diet, and we now also take supplements to make up for what is lacking in our food supply.

Eating all raw foods, never eating out, and making everything from scratch is the healthiest way to go. However, for most American families, it's just not going to happen for a myriad of reasons. Feingold is a great first step in the right direction, whether you choose to do the diet 100% or not.

Chapter 11

Contacting a Food Manufacturer

You can contact companies yourself, and I have several times. However, sometimes the customer service personnel have no clue what you are even asking. I've found it is better to e-mail the company. When I get it in writing, I'm more likely to get a more complete answer then if I talk to someone over the phone. A typical e-mail I would send might read like this:

"Hi. Our family does the Feingold Diet and we avoid artificial flavors, artificial colors (dyes), and the preservatives BHT, TBHQ, and BHA both in the foods and in the packaging that the food comes in. Could you please advise whether XYZ product contains any of these additives, and as well, whether your suppliers use any ingredients with these additives? Thank you!"

Depending upon their response, I might have to send another follow up e-mail to clarify. And I only send these e-mails out to companies where the ingredients appear clean. While I may not always get an accurate response (or as accurate as Feingold might get), surprisingly, many companies have admitted to using preservatives or another additive that we avoid. It's often the preservatives that are hidden and not listed on the ingredients. With some products like milk or juice cartons, they spray the packaging with preservatives so I will also ask about that.

When dealing with bakery items, the biggest question you want to ask is if they use any sprays containing preservatives. Here's a sample e-mail I just sent to a new gluten free bread company. I sent them an e-mail on their "Contact Us" link on their web site.

"Hi. We do the Feingold Diet and avoid preservatives like BHT, TBHQ, and BHA. I was wondering if you use any sprays on the baking pans that include these ingredients. Thank you!"

Here was their response:

"Thank you for your inquiry. The pan oil used for the non-organic bread does have TBHQ as a preservative for the oil."

I then asked about their organic bread and they said they do not use the same oil with TBHQ for their organic breads.

I called when a new cheese puff snack first came out. It was a new product so Feingold had not reviewed them yet. I read the ingredients and it looked clean. I wanted to know if it had corn syrup. The woman pulled up the ingredient list and read them to me, and said, "Nope. No corn syrup."

Thank you. I can read too. It did in fact contain corn syrup but it was listed as dextrose, and I was not familiar with all the names for corn syrup at the time (and apparently neither was she). When the product was reviewed and accepted by Feingold, it was listed as containing corn syrup.

Someone I know (not a Feingold member) contacted an accepted natural snack manufacturer to ask if one of their products contained MSG. Feingold had this specific product listed as containing MSG.

This otherwise "natural" product did not list MSG in the ingredients but she wanted to avoid MSG and wanted to make sure so she contacted the company. Here is the answer she received: "Our company does not add any manufacture MSG."

What they told her was that they do not "*add*" any "*manufacture*" MSG. However, they were using an ingredient from an outside supplier that contained MSG. They were very careful how they worded their response. This company recently admitted to removing MSG from this product which raises the question, "Why did they lie about it for so long?" It's interesting to see what lengths manufacturers will go to to conceal harmful ingredients and how difficult it can be to know for sure what truly is in a product.

Why Will Some Companies Not Fill Out Forms?

When you join Feingold, you will soon discover that there are some products that are not listed in the Feingold shopping guide but that members use without problems. Feingold has a list on their web site that shows some companies listed in black. Those companies will not fill out forms for Feingold and therefore Feingold will not list them in the shopping guide.

Why would a company not fill out forms? There are several possible reasons. It could be that they are trying to hide something. If they claim to have more natural products but really do not, they probably don't want people to know that. Or, it could be that they just don't want to use up their manpower filling out forms for Feingold. I could see this happening more often now that companies are trying to cut back on staff and save money.

Back to Nature is one company that will not fill out forms but their ingredients read clean. Many members (including our family) use their products without reactions. It just may be hard to tell if they are stage one or stage two and whether they contain any other additives that you might want to avoid like MSG or corn syrup. Please work with Feingold Back to Nature!

Occasionally, a company will fill out forms for years, and then suddenly will refuse to fill out forms. This can raise suspicions that maybe they have added an unacceptable ingredient and do not want to admit it. Frito Lay is one company that stopped filling out forms. Since the ingredients have not changed, I plan to continue using their products unless I notice a reaction in my kids.

Breyer's Natural Vanilla ice cream used to be approved but then they recently stopped filling out forms. Their ingredients did change however and some members started noticing reactions. They added tara gum and replaced the words "real vanilla" with "natural flavors." In cases where ingredients have changed and manufacturers have stopped working with Feingold, it is more likely that their ingredients are no longer acceptable.

That's why I like having access to the Feingold Members Facebook group. Even though an item is not listed, I can ask if anyone else has been using a product without reactions. I also ask if anyone knows why a specific product is not listed. If it's because a product contains artificials, then I know to avoid it.

Submitting a Product for Review

I'm hoping the information below will soon be completely outdated, but in the last nine years, this has been how products have been submitted and reviewed.

If a product you think is clean is not listed in the Feingold shopping guide, you can submit it to PIC (Product Information Committee). There's an area on Feingold's web site under Member Services where you can submit the product. Currently, you will be asked to input the product name and as much information about the product as possible (ingredients, manufacturer, your name and e-mail address, etc.). They will then contact the manufacturer (maybe).

If the product has already been reviewed or has been blacklisted (the company refuses to fill out forms), they will not contact them. You are supposed to check the list of blacklisted companies first before you submit a product. This list is located on Feingold's web site under Member Services.

If a company is listed in a certain color, it means the product is currently under review. A company can be listed as "under review" for months. Feingold waits to hear back from them. If after so many months they do not hear back, they move them to the black list for not responding and assume that they do not want to work with Feingold. Sound confusing? It is! I'm hoping they make changes soon.

Feingold recently put up a new search function on its web site. It allows members to log on and search for a product electronically. What's nice about this feature is that it also shows some of the products that are not approved under the "status" line. What's not so nice about this feature is that it requires a separate user name and password, and I always forget mine! So, if you're wondering if a product has been submitted yet or not, you could check there first.

If the manufacturer gets back to Feingold, PIC will get back to you. If the manufacturer does not respond to PIC, then PIC will not respond to you. While some manufacturers respond right away, it can take weeks or months to hear back from a manufacturer.

I'm grateful for the shopping guide and all the work that has gone in to reviewing each product so that we know what *is* clean. It's a great program and I'm all for it obviously. There are still plenty of products listed in the shopping guide that are approved.

Sometimes I feel a better use of my time is to just contact the company directly until Feingold researches a product, or if a company refuses to work with PIC. With most companies, I receive a response within a few days. I trust Feingold's information more than a direct response from a manufacturer, but if Feingold doesn't provide this information, then I will do the next best thing and contact them myself.

In my experience, the companies have disclosed the ingredients their suppliers are using as well. I'll make my decisions about whether to use a certain product based on the information that I do have. We have been on the diet for over nine years though. If you are new to Feingold, I would suggest sticking to the shopping guide in the beginning.

I sometimes list some of the products that we use without a problem on my web site. Following what we do is not the same as doing the Feingold Diet. I may list a product that I think is clean, that may not be. I am not claiming that if you use the products our family does, that you will be doing the Feingold Diet. Please do your own research as well. If you want to do the Feingold Diet, then I would follow the

Feingold shopping guide that comes with a membership. That is what we did when we first started Feingold.

My hope is that more companies will choose to work with Feingold. The ultimate goal is that more and more companies would just willingly choose to remove these harmful chemicals from our food.

Some Feingold members choose to boycott the companies that do not fill out forms or respond even though they believe their products are probably clean. Unfortunately, our family doesn't have that luxury. My kids have multiple food allergies and we are already limited as to what we can eat. But, we've also been doing the diet for nine years, and I have experience with reading labels. If there is a company that just will not fill out forms, I may choose to contact them myself and make an educated decision about whether to feed that product to my kids or not.

I included this section, not to deter anyone from purchasing a Feingold membership. It's a great program overall. It works and I'm all for it obviously. But, I just wanted to let people know that it's not a perfect program. I think some new members can get discouraged to find this information out after they've joined the program. I don't want people to get so frustrated that they give up on the entire program. It's a minor issue that can be worked around with the help of other members, and time on the program. Feingold is also continuously working to make improvements to their program.

Chapter 12

Is a Feingold Membership Worth the Money?

I struggled with this myself before buying the program. My short answer: Absolutely! This is my opinion of course, but I'll explain why. The cost of the program is currently $69 for the PDF version and $89 for the print copy (based on 2014's rates). This is your first year's fee. After the first year, you have to renew membership annually in order to get an updated shopping guide. The cost of renewal is $49 for the PDF and $59 for the printed copy. Check www.feingold.org for more complete information on what is included and the cost, as prices can change at any time.

Don't let the renewal fees deter you from trying Feingold. Give it a try for a year and then decide if you think it's worth it to continue your membership. Many members have no problem at all renewing and find that the information they are getting is invaluable as they have experienced first-hand how life changing the diet has been for their families.

It took over a year from the time I first heard about Feingold until I finally took the plunge and bought the program. I was intelligent and hard working. I thought, surely I could do this on my own and save $75. What if I spent $75 and it didn't work?

I tried to do what I could on my own. When I removed the dyes, I did notice a difference but it didn't seem to be enough. I was convinced that dyes were bad and caused issues, but I wasn't convinced that the cost of membership was really worth it.

I did more research and after reading all the pros and cons of the Feingold Diet, I weighed my options. Do I keep going like this and watch my child suffer relationally and in school, or do I give this whole diet thing a try? I prayed and decided to just go for it.

What Exactly Am I Paying For?

With a paid membership, the most important thing you will get is the annual food shopping guide and fast food guide. The foods in this guide are researched and updated continually. Feingold will send out e-mails on more popular items if there is a change, or they will just list it in their almost monthly (10 times a year) Pure Facts e-newsletter. They will send out an updated PDF guide quarterly to those that ordered the PDF. The printed shopping guide is updated once a year so you might want to use the online search tool to double check items not found in your printed guide.

Many of Feingold's workers are volunteers. They set up booths and displays at various conventions and gatherings. They print up brochures for doctors, teachers, and Feingold members and then pay for postage. They work to spread the news and educate people on the dangers of some of these harmful chemicals in our food so that families can get the help they need.

Like many of its members, these volunteers do so because their own families were helped by the Feingold Diet and they want to help others avoid the anguish they went through because of the harmful effects of certain foods. If we can spread the news, educate others, and one by one change our buying habits, we can put enough pressure on food manufacturers to change how they make and label our food. This is the ultimate goal; a world where we don't need a shopping guide and we can go to the store and buy products that are not harmful for us! Or at least clearer labeling laws that allow us to know for sure if a product contains an ingredient we want to avoid.

What About Shopping Off of Your Lists?

I have listed my personal shopping lists on my web site, and some people may think that by shopping off this list, they are doing the diet.[1] Yes and no.

These are just my personal shopping lists so you will be short changing yourself. There are many more foods that are approved that we just don't care for or cannot do because of other food allergies.

My lists can also have products listed that may have changed ingredients and are no longer approved. I don't go back and update it. I had just made a list for personal organizational purposes when I was having a baby, and decided to post it to give people an idea of what is approved on the Feingold Diet. I have also listed items that are not officially approved but look clean to me, and that we have used without noticing any reactions (after being on a clean diet for several years). If you want to make sure you are doing the diet correctly, you will have to purchase the program materials from Feingold.

Can I Do the Diet On My Own?

Yes, but I personally wouldn't want to. After reading chapter 10, you can probably understand why it's hard to do the diet on your own. So many things are not even listed on the ingredient labels. When we first started the diet, I loved having a shopping guide tell me exactly what was approved so I didn't have to go into the store and read the labels of every single product I was buying. It was a great time and sanity saver.

If you do not fully understand how the diet works, you are going to be running in circles. Literally one bite of something with red dye or another chemical could set your child off for the next two to three days. You could be going to all the trouble of watching what your child eats and then not seeing the results you would see, if you were doing the diet fully and correctly.

The other issue is salicylates. It's easy to avoid the fruits themselves, but when it is included in a natural flavor you won't know unless you contact the manufacturer. I think the biggest mistake parents unknowingly make is thinking they are doing the Feingold Diet, but not pulling stage two foods. Salicylates can have a big effect on kids and unless you take them out of the diet for at least six weeks, you won't know.

If you have a child without any major behavioral issues or if you are just trying to eat healthier, I see no problem with just trying to do your best and make healthier choices with what you know. I also realize that some people just can't afford Feingold.

Everyone can make some changes for the better. If we make a loud enough noise, maybe together we can force food manufacturers to take these chemicals out of our foods so we don't have to worry so much about it. I think raising awareness and educating other parents is key in that.

Is This Diet For Everyone?

Not everyone needs to buy the Feingold program, but I do believe that it is a great program and would benefit every family. If you have a child with issues but your family is already on a special diet and you are very up to speed on reading labels and healthy eating, you might be able to go without purchasing the program. This would be for people who cook most things from scratch, who might be on a plant-based or whole foods diet. Some of these diets already eliminate processed foods. However, the typical American family eats out frequently and eats a large volume of processed foods, so not too many people will fall under this category. Most people going into a grocery store are buying more than just fresh produce.

Today, I thank God that He gave us a child with ADHD symptoms that drove us to tears because I would have never changed the way we were eating, and never understood what goes into the foods I was feeding my kids. No parent wants to feed their kids petroleum, chemicals, and dyes that are cancer-causing, and cause behavioral and health problems. The problem is most parents don't know this or they just don't know how to feed their kids any differently.

As soon as we started the diet, I remember asking on the Feingold message board, "Why in the world didn't I hear about this on Oprah?!" I couldn't understand why this information wasn't more readily available and being broadcast on the evening news, and honestly, I was mad! My child was suffering, as was our entire family, and these food makers are well aware of the dangers of the ingredients they are using. I wanted to know why Feingold didn't market their program more.

I wish Feingold could give out their information and shopping guides for free, but then the association would cease to exist. They need some money to cover their costs and keep promoting their information to the public.

Sometimes I wish Feingold would charge more so they would have money to lobby Congress, and produce television commercials. I think everyone, and especially parents, should at least be made aware of the Feingold Diet and about what goes into our foods. I think doctors should be telling their patients about the Feingold Diet before prescribing ADHD medication. It seems that more doctors are these days, which is great. However, there are still some doctors who hold to the belief that food dyes and other additives have no effect on behavior.

For me personally, $75 was a drop in the bucket compared to what I might have spent had I not known about Feingold. I could be spending money on ADHD drugs, on numerous doctor visits (my kids stopped getting sick nearly as much once we started the diet, saving me way more than $75 on doctor visit co-pays, and over the counter medicines), on potential therapies, and on eating out (we stopped eating out as much, which wasn't an awful thing either by the way).

Before Feingold, I hated going out to eat with my kids (namely my son - sorry, honey.) He was awful! He couldn't sit still in his seat. He was constantly under the table, switching sides, running around the table, through the restaurant. I couldn't wait to get out of there. It wasn't a treat to go out to a restaurant. It was stressful and something I tried to avoid. I always thought he would outgrow this and it was just a phase at his age, but time kept passing and he was getting no better. I dreamed of the day when my kids were older and we could sit down to a meal at a restaurant in peace.

That day happened soon after we started the diet, which was such a welcome relief! I have even had strangers come up to us at a restaurant and comment on how well-behaved our kids were during the meal. We don't go out to eat very much now just because of preference really. I don't like to spend the money and health-wise, I just don't trust what kind of food they are feeding us.

But, it's nice to be able to go out and have my kids be able to behave (for the most part.) You *can* go out to eat on the diet by the way. Feingold has a Fast Food Shopping Guide that lists the fast food and chain restaurant foods that are approved. We stick to more of the basics like hamburgers, steak, and vegetables on the occasions that we do eat out.

The Feingold Message Boards

Lastly, I feel the advice and wisdom you will find on the Feingold boards (and now Facebook) from other moms who have been there is priceless! I learned way more from the other Feingold parents than I would have from the Feingold materials alone. As soon as you purchase the materials, make sure you get on the Feingold Members Facebook page right away and start reading and asking questions. This is SO important! I seriously doubt I could have done the diet correctly without being on this board frequently and asking questions. And don't worry about asking too many questions! Not a problem. Chances are, another newbie has the exact same question and is afraid to ask.

My first experience when going on the boards was one of relief. I was so relieved to find out that I was not the only one with a child like mine. I no longer felt alone. There were hundreds of other families going through the exact same thing I was, and I never realized it! I was so glad to have found them. Being able to talk to other moms and being able to post my specific questions (and I asked lots) and get immediate answers was worth way more than $75.

As well, I've learned about much more than just the Feingold Diet from the boards (and now Facebook). You will learn about healthy and natural living and about things beyond the Feingold Diet. I first learned that the GFCF diet helped kids with autism from the Feingold board. It took me a couple of years before I was ready to dive into that one, but I am thankful for the information as it quite possibly saved my son's life. His seizures are caused by a build-up of gluten, dairy, peanuts, and eggs.

Many people on the Feingold Diet are also doing other diets as well, like the GFCF diet. Feingold also recently started listing in the shopping guide whether a food is gluten or dairy free as well.

The message board found on Feingold's main web site (www.feingold.org) used to be very active and the only way to talk to other Feingold members. However, this has changed with the popularity and ease of use of Facebook. Feingold's Facebook group is much more active than the message board now.

There are two main Facebook groups, and then several other spin offs from those. The original Facebook group is called, "Feingold Association of the United States – ADHD Diet." This one is open to anyone. See the "List of Good Resources" section at the end of the book. In 2013, they started prohibiting the discussion of any brand names on this page and opened a new Facebook page for members only. This one is called "Feingold Association of the U.S. – Members Only."

The first group is more active right now as it has more members but if I have a question about a brand name, I have to post it on the Members Only page. To get access to the Members Only Facebook page, after you become a member, you have to send an e-mail to feingoldfacebook@feingold.org with your request.

There is still some valuable information to be found on the Feingold member's message board though. You can do a search on a subject and read archived posts. If I want an immediate answer to a question though, I will post it on the Facebook page.

So Is It Really Worth It?

Therapists cost at least $75 for one hour. If I had to live a couple more years with my son the way he was, I would have needed many hours of therapy! I would not have had any more kids, and my house would have been far less peaceful, and much more chaotic. So, if you ask me if Feingold is worth the cost of membership, I would have to say YES!

It reminds me of those commercials:

Price of dinner and a movie: $50
Price of a speeding ticket: $75
Price of Feingold: $69

Price of:
...the peace of mind knowing I'm feeding my kids food that is not laden with harmful chemicals

...my son getting asked on his very first play date a few weeks after starting the diet

...being able to look into my son's big beautiful eyes because he could now make eye contact and he was sitting still for the first time in his life

...not getting any more calls and notes home from the teacher for his bad behavior

...getting to know my son for who he is, and not a child controlled by the ingredients in his food

...reading my son's report cards year after year with teacher after teacher saying what a pleasure my son is to have in class

....PRICELESS!!!

Chapter 13

Is This Diet Forever?

I was watching a TV show the other night. The woman was on a bad blind date. There's a line where someone says to her, "I see your date brought along his own food." I could not stop laughing. I remember when I first started looking into the Feingold Diet. I was convinced that the diet would probably help my son but I started obsessing about all the things that I thought were going to be impossible for him to do. Going to camp, going to a friend's house, going on a date! Well, my son has gone to camp, gone to a friend's house, and some day he'll go on a date, and I don't think he'll be bringing his own food!

My dentist used to ask me every year, "Will he outgrow it?" It's not really something you outgrow. I suppose as he gets older, he is not going to react to dyes by running around in circles and having a tantrum like he did when he was four. All these chemicals do have an effect on people, whether they realize it or not. Some of those effects are visible and some of those go unnoticed for years.

However, I don't think my kids are going to be bringing their food along with them forever. Typically, the longer your diet has been clean, the better you are able to handle eating off diet on occasion. "On occasion" being the key word. The liver is cleaner and functions better when it is not constantly bombarded with toxins. We have already seen that but we also see that we definitely want and need to stay on the Feingold Diet.

I don't think it's a coincidence that in the last fifty plus years we have seen such a drastic increase in ADHD, autism, allergies, cancers and other diseases. I believe it is a direct correlation to the foods we are eating, and how much our food has changed over the last century. Toxins are one of the biggest offenses to the human body. Instead of just being exposed to toxins we are putting them directly into our bodies via the foods we eat.

Knowing what I know now, dyes, artificial flavors, and preservatives are not something I want to eat or feed to my kids. I know what they are made of and I know what it does to our bodies. I'm glad that dyes cause a reaction in my kids because if they didn't, I never would have changed the way we were eating.

People tend to look at our kids and think they are the ones with issues. However, I see it a little differently. I like to think that our kids (the ones with ADHD or autism) are the ones whose bodies are reacting to these foreign invaders just as they should. God created the body to react to toxins. It's our warning sign. Without these warning signs, we just keep on doing what we're doing, without making any changes.

They say it takes at least ten years for cancer to develop and to start showing symptoms. [1] I'm glad my kids show signs of toxicity right away. Other people can eat these foods every day but not realize what it might be doing to them silently inside. Just because they don't react in ways they can recognize as detrimental, doesn't mean it's not hurting them.

In the book, "The China Study", the authors describe cancer as developing in three stages, like grass.[1] The first stage is when seeds are spread and they start to take root under the ground. From the top of the dirt, we don't see anything, but much is going on below the surface. Over time, those seeds sprout and little blades start to appear.

Those little blades are the warning symptoms. So many people suffer from headaches and so many other ailments and have no idea why. This is our body's way of telling us that something is wrong.

More time passes, and suddenly the grass and weeds are growing wildly everywhere, between our sidewalks, in our mulch, and it is out of control for years. This is when we discover we have cancer and by that time, the seeds have taken root, and we have been feeding and letting this grow out of control.

The only way to get rid of it is through drastic measures. We kill all the cancer cells (or the grass) but what happens? If we make no changes, we will keep spreading seeds and eventually more grass grows up and we start the cycle again. I don't want to wait until it's too late to take control of my family's health.

So, is Feingold forever? I hope so! I won't have much of a say in what my kids eat when they are older and on their own. However, I hope that I have taught them well, and they choose to eat healthy for their own sake, and for the sake of their loved ones.

Is Your Son Still On the Diet?

My son is now thirteen and has been on the diet for over nine years. He still does Feingold 100 percent at home but will occasionally eat slightly off diet. We try to keep that to the weekends and when he's not in school so that he can concentrate and do his best in school. He also will eat off diet now if he goes to a friend's house. He stays away from dyes but he might eat something with preservatives or corn syrup when eating out. I think as kids get older, and especially in the teenage years, the dyes and chemicals affect their mood and emotions more.

And being in Junior High means food! Food everywhere and it's not health food. It's total junk, especially at church youth group which is kind of sad. They give out "snacks" every week at youth group which is often candy or some other dessert or junk food and then wonder why they have so many behavior problems.

The church teaches our kids not to drink or do drugs because their bodies are the temple of God. This should also apply to the foods they put into their bodies. I'm not saying they should hand out carrot and celery sticks every week, but I do think they should use much better judgment or just forego the snacks altogether.

My son will generally take the snack but only eat a small amount of it. He says that he reads the labels and that if it *only* has corn syrup, then he will eat it. I realize that as kids get older, they have to start making their own decisions about the foods they eat. I try to educate my kids on the importance of eating right.

I've told my son that he must continue to get good grades in school if I let him eat off diet every once in a while. He usually will have trouble remembering things when he eats off diet. He leaves things at school, or forgets to do some homework. He is much more clear-headed and calmer when he sticks to the diet, and more in control of his emotions.

I can always tell if he's eaten off diet. He has even noticed this for himself now. He surprised me the other day when he said he didn't want to eat out because he had an important quiz the next day that he wanted to do well on. He's also recently chosen to eat more fruits and vegetables instead of processed foods or fast food because he notices how food affects him. I'm glad that he has chosen to take control of his own health and well-being. He says when he gets older he plans to eat raw vegetables and fruit because he doesn't want to cook. OK.

I'm not condoning eating off diet just to fit in but I also realize that adolescence is a difficult time. This is how our family chooses to deal with these issues, and we have been established on the diet for several years so that also makes a difference. This may or may not be the way your family chooses to handle it. If you are new to the diet, give yourself some time to get established before deciding whether or not you want to allow your child to eat off diet on occasion. My younger kids will likely not have an option. They have serious food allergies that cannot be ignored.

The effects of artificials and preservatives can look different as a child gets older. A teenager may not show extreme hyperactivity, but he might lose focus, have trouble controlling his tongue and behavior, and get overly emotional or enraged. My son also tends to get headaches or even vomit when he eats off diet so we try to stay as close to 100 percent as possible.

When my son goes to college, he'll be on his own. I hope he sees the effects additives have on how he feels and acts and I hope he makes the decision for himself to eat healthy. I think he will. He has told me that when he gets older, he's going to try every food once, just to try it, but that he probably won't eat that stuff all the time - just every once in a while. We shall see. I hope he finds a nice Feingold girl to marry.

Chapter 14

What If the Diet Doesn't Work?

For my oldest, removing artificials and preservatives was enough. Although I'm sure there were other issues involved, it was apparent that dyes and certain additives were causing his ADHD symptoms. When we removed the dyes, artificial flavors, and preservatives, his symptoms improved greatly. When he ate off diet, his symptoms returned. So did the diet work for us? Yes! The proof was in the pudding.

Whenever there is an issue, there is a root problem or cause. In order to treat a problem, you need to find out what is causing it. That is why I'm not a fan of medication. Drugs often just mask the problem and often are not a feasible long term fix. If there is a chemical imbalance in the body, I want to know what's causing that chemical imbalance and treat it in order to see long term improvements. Dyes and other additives are chemicals that interact with the natural chemicals found in the brain which can often cause behavioral problems.[1]

If you don't see improvements on the diet, there are several possibilities as to why. In the beginning, the diet is a learning curve so give yourself some time. No one does the diet 100 percent correctly from day one.

Make sure to go on the Feingold Facebook group and ask for help. It is often helpful to post what your child has eaten the day or two prior, or what he or she typically eats to make sure you are doing the diet correctly. You might be unintentionally feeding your child something that is not approved. This is most often the case with new members who have not seen a huge difference in their child's behavior.

One bite of something not approved can cause your child to misbehave for the next couple of days. Some say if you are not doing the diet 100 percent, then you're not really doing the diet. That's not to say that any amount of effort to clean up your child's diet isn't going to be beneficial. It just means that you may not see the results you are expecting. Your child may still have the same behavior issues if you allow them to cheat here and there. There are some kids who will have improvements just by cleaning up their diet some, and there are some kids who really need to do the diet 100 percent in order to see improvements. Those are usually the kids who have been diagnosed with ADHD or some other behavioral issue.

Make sure you have switched out personal care items like toothpaste and bubble bath as those can cause issues as well because the dyes and other chemicals are being absorbed through the skin. After you switch out personal care items, look at other optional additives to avoid like corn syrup. This was huge for us and still is. Many members decide to eliminate corn syrup. You can take the chance and leave it in at first if you want. If you are not seeing improvements, then remove corn syrup and see if you notice a difference.

Keeping a diet diary is extremely helpful. Write down everything your child eats and drinks every day. I just use a notebook and start at the top and go down the page. I can fit all my kids on one page listing each child's name at the top going across. Also include any behaviors you are seeing (good or bad) and keep track of when you saw those behaviors in relation to what they have eaten.

There are a few apps out there now too which allow you to take pictures of the foods and keep your diet diary that way. They call it a photo food journal or diet tracker. Just be sure to add notes to track the behaviors you see as well.

After a while, you will start to see a pattern. You may not notice the problem food right away but keep journaling anyway. It's a bit of detective work. It is sometimes weeks later when I figure out what is causing an issue. When I look back, it becomes so clear to me which food was the problem. I have discovered several serious food allergies this way.

Next, look at removing the other additives like MSG, nitrates, etc. For us, these don't seem to cause behavioral issues, but they do give us headaches. We also avoid them for the health reasons mentioned in chapter ten. But, for some kids they are a problem.

For kids with ADHD, supplements can be helpful. Feingold suggests waiting until stage two before starting any supplements because some supplements can contain stage two ingredients or even artificials. As well, some kids can react to certain supplements, so they suggest getting to that baseline first before starting supplements. I personally think some supplements are OK to use if you know they are stage one and are ones that typically do not cause any kind of reaction in kids. But if you're using those colorful chewable vitamins advertised on TV, I'd say ditch those! Those have dyes and artificial flavors.

Getting vitamins from our food is the best way but many parents have trouble getting their kids to eat enough vegetables and other healthy foods that contain these needed nutrients. As well, the amount of nutrients in our produce today has diminished greatly over the last few decades due to the quality of our soil from poor farming practices.

So, the next best thing to eating nutrient dense food is to supplement with high quality vitamins, at least until your child's vitamin deficiencies have been addressed. Many kids, especially those with ADHD or similar issues, have specific vitamin deficiencies. I have a post on my web site entitled, "10 Supplements for ADHD." [2] Check with your doctor before starting any supplements.

There are many supplements that have been shown to be very helpful for kids with ADHD, as many of these kids have the same deficiencies. Along with a toxic diet, vitamin deficiencies are also a contributing factor to ADHD behaviors. But, the first rule of order is to get the diet under control. Adding supplements alone may help some, but improvements will likely be overshadowed by a poor diet.

I had my children's vitamin levels tested through my holistic doctor and he advised us on which supplements to take and the suggested dosages. Cleaning up the diet will also help with vitamin deficiencies. When you reduce the amount of toxins going into the body, the body can go after the real toxins and offenders like bacteria, yeast, parasites, and precancerous cells which may be feeding off of all those vitamins and nutrients that your child's body needs. Our kids often benefit from taking supplements which make up for those deficiencies.

Yeast overgrowth is another common underlying cause for ADHD as well as autism. Doing Feingold stage one and cutting down on sugar can help with yeast. There are a lot of supplements for yeast as well. I did a post on how we treat yeast in our house. [3] See the References section at the end of this book

If Feingold does not seem to be working, some people consider removing gluten and/or dairy. I say, try to do Feingold stage one 100 percent first before trying GFCF. Sometimes those considering GFCF are not doing the Feingold Diet fully. Going gluten and dairy free is a lot harder than just doing Feingold. If you only need Feingold, it will be much easier on you and your child. This is not to say that removing gluten and dairy might be beneficial to your child. I believe that gluten and dairy are not the best things for our bodies.

However, if you are only trying GFCF because you want to correct a behavioral problem like hyperactivity, I think it is better to try Feingold 100 percent first. If you try to dive right in to a modified Feingold Diet *and* a GFCF diet, you may get very overwhelmed and give up on both diets. For some people, their children have more severe issues and medical concerns (like constant stomachaches, headaches, ear infections, digestive difficulties, seizures, etc.), so doing both diets may be the best option.

It is often the kids who have issues beyond just ADHD such as autism, or who have digestive issues, who find a GFCF diet very helpful. My younger kids have digestive issues which may be caused by Leaky Gut Syndrome. [4] When kids with a leaky gut eat gluten or dairy, it causes an opiate reaction. The kids will get hyper and giddy, almost like they are on drugs or drunk when they eat gluten and dairy.

Then the next day, if they don't have gluten or dairy again, they go into withdrawal and are extremely moody and ravishingly hungry. Their bodies are trying to get that gluten and dairy fix again. I can attest to this as I do GFCF as well. It's not fun so we try to stay on the GFCF diet 100 percent to avoid withdrawal symptoms.

Why not just let them eat gluten and dairy every day then? Because it causes many other unwanted behaviors and symptoms like constipation, diarrhea, bloated belly, seizures (for my youngest son), hyperactivity, dark circles under the eyes, runny nose, sluggishness, loss of energy, suppression of the immune system, headaches, and much more.

Symptoms are not the same for everybody but for certain kids, a GFCF diet is very helpful. The topic of gluten and dairy is another big one. I will discuss gluten and dairy more in another book in the future.

There are many other diets that eliminate even more foods and additives, avoiding things like GMO's and most processed foods. I believe an organic, raw foods diet is probably the best way of eating. The problem is getting your kids to eat raw, finding the time to make all raw foods, and living in an area of the country where organic produce might not always be readily available.

I'm not saying you should avoid a raw foods diet. If you can do it, go for it. Many people do. It's my goal to get there some day. In the meantime, we add as many raw foods into our diet as possible. We dehydrate fruits and vegetables and I'm currently looking into juicing (trying to find some good stage one recipes that my kids will actually drink.) I also like Dr. Joel Fuhrman's nutritarian diet approach (eliminating almost all processed foods and eating foods high in nutrients like greens, veggies, nuts, beans, and berries). [5] However, a nutritarian diet is hard to implement when you are Feingold stage one as well.

Does Feingold Help Kids With Autism?

For my younger kids, one with autism, Feingold alone was not enough. The Feingold Diet was certainly one of the factors required for my daughter's improvement, but we took things further than just Feingold. I had read about the GFCF diet on the Feingold board for a couple of years. I knew it helped some kids with autism, but I thought, "My daughter would starve if we did GFCF. That's all she eats."

I had no idea how to start GFCF so I just never tried it. When my younger son started having seizures, I was forced to give the diet a try. We noticed improvements right away. Gone were the runny noses, stomachaches, dark circles under the eyes, and constipation. And the seizures stopped! My daughter's energy levels skyrocketed and she no longer complained of needing to sit in the stroller or shopping cart (at age four). She started becoming more aware of her surroundings and her speech and cognitive abilities improved.

I suspected my daughter might have autism so we started seeing a DAN! (Defeat Autism Now!) doctor around the same time. He did some tests including a food allergy test. We started supplements and treated for yeast overgrowth. We tweaked her diet some more and saw even more improvements.

Dyes and chemicals exacerbate autistic symptoms, but additives alone are not the sole cause of autism. Toxins and methylation issues (the body's ability to rid the body of toxins) are one major cause of autism, so reducing the amount of toxins going in to the body via food is definitely a necessary step.

Feingold often helps reduce some autistic behaviors such as tantrums and meltdowns. Salicylates are often a problem for kids with autism.

My daughter never had issues with hyperactivity. She had hypotonia (low muscle tone) so she was never running around like her older brother. She does have difficulty concentrating and focusing in school though, as is common with kids on the spectrum.

As kids with autism improve and heal through biomed (using tests, diet, and supplements with the help of a holistic doctor), they often are left with "only" ADHD symptoms. For kids with autism, this means they are recovering.

Kids with autism have much more complex issues than kids with just ADHD. Kids on the autism spectrum often have immune system dysfunctions, yeast and bacteria overgrowth, malabsorption issues, food allergies, digestive problems, an inability to remove toxins from the body leading to toxic overload, and much more.

A child with autism is probably not going to lose their autism diagnosis as sometimes happens with kids diagnosed with ADHD when they go on the Feingold Diet. However, Feingold is definitely helpful and necessary. Some kids on the spectrum do see big improvements with Feingold stage one. We started Feingold when my daughter was eighteen months old so I have no clear "before" and "after" to see how the diet affected her.

So, to answer the question, does Feingold help kids with autism? I would say yes, it is definitely a necessary first step and you will likely see some improvements, but I believe that more is needed to properly address all of the root causes of autism.

Other Issues

Obviously, there are also other issues that come into play with ADHD-like symptoms too. Some kids act up because of something going on in their lives. There might be problems at home or they might be dealing with some kind of emotional pain. Not everything can be blamed on diet, but food is a good place to start. I've been amazed over and over again at how food affects behavior and physical ailments. If my kids ever act up, the first thing my family will ask is, "What did they eat?" Their behavior is not always caused by something they ate though; sometimes they are just acting like normal children.

For some kids inactivity and electronic overload play a role in ADHD-like behaviors. We've all heard that video games and too much television is bad for kids. I believe it. We had to get rid of the Power Rangers movies my son had when he was three. He was noticeably more violent after watching them.

Many kids with ADHD are addicted to video games. I plan to research this more someday. It's hard for parents (myself included) to tell their hyperactive kids to stop playing video games because it provides the parents a much needed break. For the kids, I think it feels like therapy to them.

In the summer, my kids are outside playing a lot. They tend to behave better when they are able to get outside and get some exercise. I wish we lived in a warmer climate because they are not able to get out and run around in the winter in the Midwest.

So, try to get your kids to do some more physical activity as well. Sometimes my kids will set up an obstacle course in our house using chairs, pillows, blankets, the beds, the mini trampoline, etc. Then they run all through the house running through the obstacle course. They think this is big fun.

If you've tried all of the above suggestions and the diet has not worked, you can move on from there to investigate other possible issues. I personally would not ditch the whole diet, but I would see what other things I could do on top of removing chemicals from their food. Purchasing the Feingold program is not going to solve all your problems. Feingold is not some magic bullet that works just by buying it. It is a helpful guide and support system but you still have to do the work and make wise decisions on what you choose to feed your kids.

Also, some behavior issues have to do with disciplining and parenting styles. There is a Feingold member and mother of six who has a signature line that says, "Remember, Feingold won't give you a perfect child. It will give you a child who responds correctly to loving, consistent discipline." So true!

There's a saying, "Christians aren't perfect, just forgiven." For Feingold that would be, "Our kids aren't perfect, just chemical free!" My kids are far from perfect. I think that makes them pretty normal. I have yet to meet a perfect child or a perfect parent, perfect diet or not.

Kids are often getting into trouble and being reprimanded which can affect their self-esteem. I heard a pastor say how he tells his kids that he loves them no matter what they do. When my son was about six, I told him one night that there was nothing he could do to make me stop loving him. I would love him no matter what. He turned around and gave me a hug. Aww.

I had the same conversation with my daughter one night before bed. She thinks very literally. As I was laying there in the dark, I felt a big fist in my face. Ouch! She punched me! I said, "What was that for?" She smiled and said, "Do you love me now?" Not quite the response I was looking for!

I know I've introduced a lot of big topics above without going in to much detail. I just wanted to make people aware of some of the things "beyond Feingold" that might be helpful. I plan to write another book detailing out how to go about starting a supplement regimen, treating for yeast, and if a gluten and dairy free diet is right for your child, and how to start that. But for now, the Feingold Diet is where you want to start. Once you have that established, you can start to look into other things. We all want our kids helped right away, but it's wise to take things one step at a time.

If all of these things don't work, don't give up! Give yourself a few months to learn the diet and make sure you are not feeding your child harmful additives inadvertently. Keep a diet diary and watch for patterns. If you keep searching for answers, you will eventually find them. Or, you might just need to take things a step further. I hope you come to realize that eating a diet free of harmful chemicals is healthier for your child regardless.

Chapter 15

Feingold Success Stories

OK, so we just talked about what to do if the diet doesn't work, so I thought it'd be a good time to hear some Feingold success stories! I think the number one question parents want to know is: "Does it really work?" Here is what a few Feingold parents had to say.

Feingold works! So thankful to have my 4-year old daughter able to concentrate and sit still - hold eye contact even! It was tough at first but completely worth it. It is now just a way of life and we are all better for it!

Amanda, LA

We are three weeks in on stage one and my son is like a completely different kid. He is calmer, more in control, expressing himself better, and even his tantrums (he's 5) are different. Normally, he's throwing himself on the floor and crying uncontrollably for 30+ minutes. Now, he's barely crying, talking about why he's upset, and rebounding quickly. I am astonished at this change.

Jessica, WV

When I actually sit down and contemplate our lives now compared to two years ago, I am still amazed! I recall watching the documentary, "Generation Rx" and "Frontline: The Medicated Child." Both programs literally brought me to tears. It was just the realization of what society would have us do to our children. While some children may need those drugs, the VAST majority do not! Now, every year when I renew membership, I see it as a privilege. I look forward to it. This diet has made a day and night difference in the quality of life for each member of our family! Thank you Feingold!!!

Peggy, WI

Oh, the PEACE!!!!! I could cry - this is so fantastic!! My daughter and I are both MED FREE!!!!! I had been misdiagnosed as having Bipolar Disorder in 2011 (meds for that only helped for two weeks), had inconclusive results on my ADHD testing last summer, and just diagnosed with anxiety and depression (that weren't responding well to any of the meds I was put on). I did end up getting an ADHD diagnosis from my Psych recently and was put on Vyvanse, which worked longer than any of the previous meds, but I had started getting irritable again even after a recent dosage increase (less than five weeks of relief was all I got). But now??! I'm so nice and patient it's almost scary!! I keep telling my husband, "I'm just so 'chill' right now", lol. Nothing bothers/irritates me like before, and I don't have to "white knuckle" my way through life anymore!! I don't have any weird OCPD issues anymore! So much better than being on any pill. My daughter is so responsible, calm, thoughtful, and just a JOY! And all of this has happened in the NINE DAYS since starting Feingold!

Rachel, WV

I put my son on meds which caused severe tics, aggression, detachment, and suicidal thoughts...that's when I said enough! I researched for two days alternative treatments for ADHD and found Feingold. I am so grateful now for getting my son back. Tics are almost gone. He has returned to the sweet, affectionate boy I had before the meds and he is able to complete his school work. We have now been eating clean, unprocessed foods for a year and I couldn't be happier. It changed our lives!

Elizabeth, CA

My 4-year old boy was tagged as strong-willed, red-headed stubborn, too smart for his brain to process correctly, stuck in the terrible two's, etc. Fortunately, my kid acted this way regardless of who he was with, so I knew in my heart it wasn't parenting/ discipline related. My son was the perfect baby until he reached ten months and started eating "normal" foods. From then on he had repeated ear infections, unexplained stuffy nose and rashes.

We were always walking on egg shells with him because we never knew when he was going to act perfectly and when something like getting a drop of water on his sleeve might send him into a two hour long violent tantrum. Finally I read that it wasn't normal for a toddler to keep crying after you offered them what they wanted. My toddler didn't tantrum because he didn't get his way. I realized that he wasn't normal.

I found Feingold on a comment on an article about food dye and realized that the food was causing his episodes. His "episodes" resembled seizures and resulted in so many physical and emotional injuries. Following Feingold, our longest crying spurt has been ten minutes and no one got hurt!!! Feingold saved our family!! I had a hunch for three years that something food related/ environment was causing his issues, but Feingold gave us the tools and resources to prove that. We will be forever grateful!

Amy, MI

My son was diagnosed ADHD almost seven years ago. Because we went on the Feingold program, he never had to go on meds, and went from failing 3ʳᵈ grade and getting kicked out of private school, to being in the Honors program just two years later. I always knew there was a beautiful, brilliant, kind, happy boy in there and Feingold helped us find him. The beginning was hard, detoxing and adjusting, but MUCH less hard than dealing with a child that can't learn, can't behave, can't control his emotions and hates himself for doing all those things! I decided it couldn't hurt to try the program and if it helped, go from there, but it was all he ever needed. The ONLY "treatment" we did was get him on the program – changed his diet, eliminated all other chemicals, personal products, cleaning, air fresheners, perfumes, etc. We also have to watch his exposure to gas fumes, ink (on skin), and markers. But it is all so worth it. It changed our lives!! And most importantly, his. It has given him the future he wants and deserves.

Melanie, DE

My husband and I are the lucky parents of two wonderful children with our daughter who is seven and our son who is five. My son has always been highly energetic and fun, sometimes to the point of all of our complete exhaustion. In March of 2012, I was at a play date with a friend that happened to be a physician that suggested that my son might have ADHD. Not that I didn't suspect something was wrong. It is just that I didn't want there to be something wrong. We just lived most of our lives outdoors to cope with his high energy expenditure needs. However, I did keep him away from food dyes because Lord help us if he ingested a food dye. I would have to peel him off the walls. And isn't a little brother supposed to torment his older sisters? Don't little boys sometimes throw screaming tantrums on the floor?!? I took her advice and went to see a specialist that stated, "This is a very obvious case of

ADHD." *He stated that when we were ready for medication, my son would be a good candidate. Not wanting to take the route of medicating his symptoms but finding a cause, I began researching other routes and did decide to take him to play therapy in the meantime.*

It was four weeks into play therapy when my research led me to Dr. Feingold's website and I quickly ordered the information. I began the lifestyle change as a skeptic, but I was ASTOUNDED when two days after changing his eating habits my son was a completely different kid. When I say completely different I mean this is who he was always meant to be but his body was so hypersensitive to salicylates, food dyes, and preservatives that the chemicals were not allowing him to be himself.

One week after I started him on the Feingold diet, we had our fifth play therapy session and I didn't say a word to the therapist about the diet changes. When the session was over, the therapist came out with my son and asked, "Did you put him on medication because this is not the same little boy I have been visiting with?" I excitedly told him about the dietary changes and he was very accepting and took all my information about it. He stated that he would start recommending this to other clients.

So many times I thought, "I know I am a good mom. I feed him mostly organic meals with fruits (majority were berries) and veggies, so why is this happening?" The hardest part was when we would visit family that live twelve hours away and they would give a lot of unsolicited advice such as, "Whip him. You aren't being tough enough. He's a brat. Can't you control him?" I am loving, patient, and I discipline him appropriately so why do I feel like he is slipping through my fingers and why do so many people think I am such a slacking parent?

I now have the proof that we are good parents and that it was the chemicals that were causing the chaos on his little central nervous system. We are strictly a Feingold family now and I am very happy to report that he is a wonderful, loving, and sweet little boy.....although he is sometimes a typical naughty little five year old.

Symptoms before Feingold:

1. Quick tempered

2. Always in a constant state of motion

3. Constantly picking fights with his sister or other little children

4. Very hard to reason with.

Symptoms after Feingold: None - just normal mischief!

Ami, TX

My 5-year-old has been on the Feingold diet for almost a year. I was a little unsure of how it was working until I gave her a pickle one day (yellow 5). She was back to "mad woman" status. Today, her aunt picked her up from preschool. She came home completely nuts! Stomping on toys, jumping on and off of furniture, not listening.... She told me later that her aunt (who knows better!) had gotten her an ice cream cone that was blue. Grrr!!! I KNOW that it is this crap that they put in "kid food" that is resulting in these poor kids being medicated without reason. Feingold is the way to go! I had forgotten how looney she used to act until I see it when she has a reaction.

Bethany, TX

We started the Feingold diet about three months ago when my son was diagnosed with Tourette's. The diagnosis and diet are very overwhelming but I'm doing the best I can.

Before I started the diet I didn't really believe in all of the food sensitivities I was hearing about. Gluten? Really? That's made up! Food dye...who cares!!!!! Well fast forward to a Tourette's diagnosis and I was willing to try anything.

I started the diet hoping just to get my sweet calm boy back. I did! His tics also went down by 3/4. If that didn't make me a believer the introduction of raspberries did. I gave them to him one day. The next day he woke up with his three regular tics and three NEW tics added to the mix. His behavior was out of control. I had never seen him like that. It took him three days to detox. OFF OF RASPBERRIES!!!!! Who would have thought?! I fed him mixed berries almost every day before we started the diet.

I would be lost without this diet. It's amazing what an effect food has on us.

Marlene, IL

Chapter 16

Encouragement & Advice for Newbies

When researching the Feingold Diet, many parents feel overwhelmed and wonder if they can do this diet or not. You're not alone. Many of us have been there. You are the one that God put into your child's life and He put you there for a reason. You *can* do this. Philippians 4:13 says, "I can do all things through Christ who gives me strength." [1]

When our family first started Feingold, I was working at my parents' trucking company as the Office Manager. I hired and fired people. I ordered the office supplies and set up procedures so that everything ran smoothly. I solved problems and put out "fires" every day.

I was successful at work and I knew how to make things run well, but at home it was a different story. I looked at the state of my child and I made the decision to put my family first. It wasn't as important how well I did at work and how far up the ladder I climbed. If I could manage an office, I should be able to manage my child and my home just as well, if not better.

I didn't quit my day job (not till later anyway), but I decided I needed to put my energy and focus on my family. I knew there wasn't much glory or appreciation in being a mom and I wouldn't be getting any special recognition or a "Mom of the Month" award, but I believed that God was calling me to bring all of my talents and abilities I used at work into my home. I wanted to live out Colossians 3:23 in my home -

"Whatever you do, work at it with all your heart, as working for the Lord, not for men." [2] So much of what we do as moms behind the scenes goes unnoticed, but not entirely. God sees, and it *is* important.

I Corinthians 10:31 says, "So whether you eat or drink, or whatever you do, do it all for the glory of God." [3] It's funny that this verse mentions eating and drinking. My takeaway is this: I will strive to do everything I do to bring glory to God. I made the decision to do my best to take care of my son and to help him live a life that glorified God.

If you are going to be successful at something, it helps to first determine what your motivation is. For some, that motivation may be avoiding those intimidating phone calls from teachers threatening to kick your child out of class if they don't start behaving. It may be remembering all the times your child has acted up and caused chaos in your home. It may be striving to keep your child off ADHD medication. It may be watching your child struggle with friendships. Whatever it is, that is what's going to motivate you to keep going when it seems tough and when you think you can't do this. And of course, for many parents, it is simply for the love of their child. Many parents would do anything to help their child.

For me, it is a combination of things. I believe this diet is what's best for my whole family. I believe that it brings honor to God to treat our bodies as temples and living sacrifices. I know that avoiding dyes and harmful additives may offend some people. Extended family members may tell you that you should just let your kids eat whatever they want because everyone else feeds their kids dyes and it's easier.

My goal is not to do what's easiest in life, but what is best. My objective is to please God, not others. Some people just don't know any better. As Maya Angelou says, "When you know better, you do better."[4]

If you mess up or don't do the diet perfectly, don't worry. Nobody's perfect. There may be a day when your child eats off diet for whatever reason. Don't think that the world is over. Tomorrow is another day. Just start again the next day and learn from your mistakes.

If after reading this book you're thinking this is too much and you don't think it's the right fit for your family - that's OK too. Some families know that with work and their family's lifestyle, they wouldn't be able to do the diet 100 percent. I hope you've at least become more aware of how food can affect behavior. I think everyone can make better choices and there may come a time later when you are ready or need to start the diet.

I'm not out to promote the Feingold Diet to the exclusion of everything else. I just want to share our experiences and offer hope. The Feingold Diet worked for my son who had ADHD symptoms and other issues. For me it was worth all the extra effort I had to put forth in the beginning. After being on the diet for over nine years now, I can't say that it's a whole lot of extra effort to just do Feingold. We do GFCF plus a whole lot more and I am cooking for four kids. Is there a lot of work and effort in doing that? Definitely!

My goal in writing about the Feingold Diet is that more parents are made aware of the diet, especially if they have a child with ADHD or similar issues. I want parents to know that there are other options besides medication. And I can't say it enough - I want manufacturers to stop putting these harmful chemicals into our food, especially in foods marketed to our children. Until we make noise about these harmful additives, and our shopping patterns affect their bottom line, they are not going to change.

As moms, we need to educate other moms. As parents, we need to contact our schools and request the celebration of birthdays via brightly colored junk food be eliminated and other celebrations be toned down. We need to contact manufacturers via e-mail or Facebook and tell them we want these harmful additives taken out of our food. Alone, each of us only has one voice, but we need to use whatever influence we do have, and together we can make a difference.

Any Advice For Newbies?

Yes! As soon as you sign up for membership, go on Facebook and request to join the Feingold members Facebook page. Go on and start reading and ask lots and lots of questions! Don't be shy. Honestly, I'm on so many different Facebook groups that I don't pay much attention to the names of those asking the questions. So, not many are going to notice if you ask a million questions.

Also keep in mind that there is a high likelihood that another newbie has the exact same question. And you're helping Feingold improve the program. If newbies are asking the same question over and over, then they know what they can do or change to make the program easier for newbies.

While Feingold is technically only about removing certain chemicals, some of the members of Feingold are highly educated on healthy living and eating that extends way beyond just Feingold. I've learned a lot from other Feingold members and I think you will find it to be good therapy. It's so nice to know that you are not alone in this journey. I'm positive I would not have been able to do Feingold correctly without being on the board (and now Facebook) frequently and asking questions.

And expect to feel overwhelmed at first. Every single one of us did too. It gets easier. Just take things one day at a time and try not to get stressed out over it. If you mess up, don't worry. With every failure, you are one step closer to success.

You don't have to do this all at once either. If you need time to read and go shopping and get some recipes together, do it. It won't kill your kids to wait another week or two to officially start the diet. It takes time to make things and stock your freezer. There is no Feingold food police that's going to show up at your door if your kids eat off diet. It's your family and you get to decide what to feed them.

I think we're the hardest on ourselves. Sometimes we need to give ourselves a break. If you get so overwhelmed that you just want to give up on the whole thing, don't. Just step back and take a break. It's better to do the diet somewhat than not at all. Keep reading and trying new foods and recipes and when you're ready to start the diet fully, then do so.

Keeping treats on hand helps in the beginning too. Your kids won't feel so deprived of their favorite foods if they are distracted by new treats. While this isn't the healthiest route, it's effective and it's only short term. Reward your kids with a dessert or something else if they try a new meal or food.

The biggest thing I've learned is "be prepared." We never left the house without snacks and juice or water. I even had candy or gum in my bag, just in case it was needed. You never know when someone's going to offer your kid something. We got in a car accident once and the firefighter offered my son a sucker. Good thing I had a natural one on hand to swap out. Keep an open communication with your child's teacher to find out when they are having treats at school.

Stage one can be hard to get through but remind yourself and your kids that stage one may not be forever. And above all, *don't give up!* You *can* do this!

Chapter 17

Other Frequently Asked Questions

Do You Have Any Association With Feingold?

No; other than the fact that I have been a member continuously for the last nine years. I don't make any money if you purchase their program.

I sincerely enjoy helping others and as a Christ follower, it is what I am called to do. "Love your neighbor as yourself." Mark 12:31b [1]

I feel like it would be selfish for me to keep this information to myself. The Feingold Diet helped us so much. I'm more than happy to help spread the word and help struggling families. As well, there have been many moms who have helped me out along the way, taking the time to answer my many questions. I am honored to do the same for someone else.

What If My Husband's Not On Board?

If your husband's not supportive, you're not alone! Many husbands are not in the beginning. It's usually the moms who are dealing with the misbehavior day in and day out and then doing all the research.

If it's a money issue, I would pray about it. Maybe decide with your husband that if and when God provides the money to buy the program, then you will do it. Have a garage sale, sell some items online, or if you come into some unexpected money, use it to purchase the program.

Feingold doesn't have to be expensive. You can make things from scratch if you can't afford the prepackaged items. My stance was if God wanted me to do this, then He was also capable of providing.

I believe it's often harder for dads to admit that there is a problem, especially in boys. They want to think they are just being boys. Or maybe they think it will be too much work for their wives. Or they don't like the idea of their child being different and having to bring their own food places.

While their concerns are valid, they need to understand that dealing with their child the way they are is so much *more* work for their wives. The emotional toll is worse. Having a child that is under control is going to make mom so much happier. And you know what they say, "If mom's happy, everyone's happy."

Moms are usually the main ones responsible for the care of the children, especially if they are a stay at home mom. Taking care of the kids is their job. What if a woman one day went in to her husband's place of work, sat down at his desk, and just started doing his job and making decisions for the things he is responsible for? She has not spent the same amount of hours on this job as her husband has and the people under him might suffer from her decisions based on her lack of experience on the job.

Her husband would go back to his job the next day and have to deal with the decisions his wife made. I see this the same way. Husbands should let their wives do their jobs. Of course I'm not saying all husbands are clueless and are not involved in their children's lives.

Husbands should be involved but the reality is that most moms spend more time child rearing.

Some moms have told me their husbands won't let them do the diet. To me, being a leader means listening to your wife's concerns. I think if husbands want to be the one responsible for making such a decision, they should spend the same amount of time researching this diet as their wives.

If after that, they still think it's a bad idea, I say they should express their opinion but still support their wife if she decides she wants to do it. I personally don't believe that submission means outright obedience, no matter what. I think both spouses are equal and the husband's stance should take precedence when it involves bigger issues, especially of spiritual significance.

As a wife, it's frustrating if your husband's not on board because you are put under more pressure to make the diet work. I would pray about it but ultimately I personally believe in doing what is best for my children as I am responsible to God for how I take care of my children. Does that mean I would go out and purchase the program despite my husband's request that I not? No, it means I would do my best to do the diet on my own and pray that God would change his heart.

It's much easier though if you can get your husband on board before you purchase the program. Husbands can sometimes feel left out. Try to involve them as much as possible. Watch some of the documentaries listed at the end of this book together. Let your husband order or pick out approved candy or treats for the kids. Then let him be the one to give the candy to the kids. Give your husband a list of what is approved so he can do some of the shopping. If you order the PDF version, you can send him a copy so he has it on his phone.

I made one shelf in our pantry that was just for my son. That way, anyone in our house (including babysitters and grandparents) would know which foods my son could have.

There is one Feingold mom who pinned every food her kids liked and could have on to her Pinterest board, along with notes such as "stage one" or which store the item could be found at. This way, her husband has a picture of each food and there is no confusion as to what their child could or could not have. This is ingenious! I just started some Feingold boards myself. (www.pinterest.com/allnaturalmom4). This is a great way to keep ex-spouses up to date on acceptable foods as well.

Try to get your husband to read something – anything. Relay what you have learned. Whatever you do, try to get them to support your decision. It will make it easier for everyone. Or, see if he'll give it a short trial run if he says no (without grilling you if you don't see huge results at first).

Most husbands are skeptical in the beginning, but often times, once they see the results, they become believers. Don't expect it to happen right away, but it often does happen, so don't lose hope.

And for all those husbands who do support their wives...YOU ROCK!!! Your wives are very lucky! We would love to see more of you on the Feingold Facebook group. Your perspective is very helpful, especially when women are trying desperately to get their husbands on board with the diet. And, the group will help you understand your wife's perspective a little more, and she will love you for it! This should be a team effort.

I know this can be a very touchy issue for some couples. I'm not giving any marital advice. You know your husband and your situation best, so do what you feel is best for your individual family. These are just my humble (or not so humble) opinions.

Should I Buy the Printed Shopping Guide or the PDF?

If you're new to Feingold, you might find the printed copy a little easier to use. However, the PDF version has been gaining a lot of popularity for a few reasons. With the increase in the use of I-Pads, smart phones, and tablets, people are finding the PDF version to be really convenient. You can have your shopping guide handy when out at the store and quickly look up an item. I recently renewed with the PDF for the first time, and I love it! It is so much quicker and more convenient to look up an item as I always have my phone on me.

The PDF version is updated every quarter so you'll get four updates per year via an e-mail. With the printed copy, you only get one copy for the year until you renew again. The printed copy does get updated every quarter as well. However, depending on when you originally purchased the program, the information may not be completely up to date.

For example, I purchased the program in February, 2005. It was likely last updated in November or December of 2004 for the 2005 book printing. The following February, I renewed my subscription and got the 2006 book. So, with the PDF, you will get the most up to date information if there are any changes in approved products or ingredients.

You won't be left in the dark on updates though if you purchase the printed copy. When there are changes to the shopping guide, Feingold will note this in their almost monthly (10 times per year) e-newsletter, called Pure Facts. It's usually a pretty long list of both stage one and stage two items. If you are vigilant and have the time, you can hand write these changes into your hard copy, or at least note the products that you use often.

Past archived newsletters can also be viewed on Feingold's web site but the current years can only be seen by current members. The newsletter is filled with some really good information and is really educational.

If you want a printed hard copy, you can just print yourself one. I would suggest printing it out two-sided to save on paper. And some newbies print only stage one. Then you can three-hole punch the papers and put them into a binder. Now you have the best of both worlds. Feingold says it is about the same cost to purchase a hard copy from them and have both the PDF and a book, but it just depends on your printer I guess.

When you buy the PDF version, you are able to download the PDF within 24 hours usually. I've heard some people say they got it within a few hours, and others within a day or two. It's an e-mail that Feingold sends you. If you purchase the hard copy, it takes about two weeks to get your shopping guide and other materials. That's a long time to wait, especially in this day and age. You do have the option of paying extra to have the materials overnighted to you though.

Another reason I like the PDF: it's cheaper! The PDF is currently $20 cheaper than the printed copy. And with the PDF, no more having to look up stage one and stage two! I can't stand doing this with the printed copy. When you search for an item on the PDF, using Adobe Acrobat, I just have to hit the right arrow button, and within a few seconds, it shows me the stage two items. No more looking back and forth through the book to look at both stage one and stage two items, which are separated into two different sections of the book. Also, it can sometimes be hard to find an item in the book if you don't know what it was classified under. I've missed some approved items only because I was looking in the wrong place in the book.

This can happen with the PDF as well, but I've had success with a few tweaks. You might just have to try a couple different ways to look up an item. For example, I was looking for an approved cereal. I input "cereal" and it brought up cereal bars. It scans the PDF and looks for that exact word. I've found the easiest way is to input the name brand of the product I'm looking for.

And what if you've already purchased the hard copy and you want to upgrade to the PDF? Currently, that'll cost you $25. If you purchase the PDF, and then want a hard copy, that will cost you $28.50 as of 2014. Or you can just wait until your renewal and get the PDF version then.

Why purchase the printed copy? If you're not comfortable with technology or don't have any of these electronic devices, the hard copy works just fine too. I actually have always purchased the hard copy because I like to have something in my hand to highlight and mark up. As a newbie, if I had both the PDF and hard copy available to me, I know I would have done better with the hard copy.

However, when somebody mentioned that you could just print off a copy, I decided to renew with the PDF this year. If you're worried about losing your PDF (if your computer crashes, etc.), just e-mail your PDF to yourself so you always have it. You can also e-mail Feingold, and they will send you a new link. I like having both the PDF and the printed out copy in case I have any trouble with the search feature on my phone. I also often just ask on the Feingold members Facebook group if I have trouble finding an item on my PDF.

On your tablet, you can open up and save the PDF using iBook or a similar app for your device. I used Adobe Acrobat on my iPhone. From my e-mail on my phone, I opened up the PDF, then saved it to Adobe Acrobat. Make sure you have the most recent version of whatever app you use if you haven't upgraded it in a while.

This then allows you to do a search for items within the PDF. If you need help doing this, just post on the Facebook page and someone can walk you through it. It can be a little different for each device. You can highlight and make notes. However, I'm thinking once you get the updated PDF the following quarter, you will not be able to keep your highlights, so just keep that in mind. The PDF also allows you to share your shopping guide with your spouse which can be really helpful for grocery shopping.

When downloading it to your computer, save it to your computer first. I put mine on my desktop. Then when you want to search for an item, you will use control+F. (Think "find.")

If you purchase the hard copy, you also have the option of going on Feingold's web site and looking up an item there too. This was implemented in 2013. It's similar to having the PDF version, but it allows those without the PDF, to go online and look up an item. This is nice if you can't find your shopping guide or you are not at home but have access to a computer. You do have to be a current member to get access to this and you will have to input a password.

So which form of the shopping guide is better? It really depends on what you are comfortable with. If you're not good with technology or don't have a smart phone or tablet, you will probably want to go with the book. If it is your first time ordering the program, some people like having the book in hand to thumb through. This isn't a bad idea as they will send you several documents to read through, not just the shopping guide. If you're new to the program and order the PDF, I would suggest printing yourself out a copy to have as well. Or, if you have the money, you could order both the PDF and the printed copy.

Is There an App for That?

Many members would love to see an app where you could just scan an item at the grocery store and it would tell you if it's Feingold acceptable or not. I'm thinking this would be a long way's off though as it would require a lot of money and manpower to get it set up and keep it maintained, but it would be so awesome!

There is an app called NxtNutrio, Healthy Diet and Gluten-Free, Allergy, GMO Finder. Lifetime Fitness is currently offering this app free to its members under the app name LifeCafe Healthy Pantry. Contact your local Lifetime Fitness if you are a member for more information.

You can scan a product and it will tell you if it contains dyes, gluten, dairy, soy, GMO's, MSG, high fructose corn syrup, and a few other things. It also tells you why a particular ingredient is bad for you. This is a really cool app. I'm hoping they expand it to include even more things like corn syrup. Some products are not in their system but it's easy to send the product to them to have them research it. If this company paired up with Feingold, I would love it! Hopefully over time, more apps will come out like this one.

This app is a nice supplement to Feingold but it is not the same as doing Feingold. Feingold tells you if an item is stage one or stage two, and they also do a more in depth research of products to find any hidden ingredients or harmful chemicals used in the packaging or by a company's supplier. But, it's helpful to see when a product does for sure contain an ingredient you want to avoid if you are not experienced at reading labels.

Some members would also like to see the shopping guide available as an app instead of a PDF file. Hopefully someday it will be. But as of 2014, it is not.

Do I Need To Purchase Any of the Other Items For Sale?

When purchasing the program, you basically just need to purchase either the PDF version or the paperback books which are currently listed at $69 or $89. Below that, Feingold offers some other items for sale. These are all optional and you don't need any of them to do the diet. They are basically extra reading materials.

I have not purchased the cookbooks so I can't say if they're any good or not. However, all of the recipes listed in the cookbooks are also listed in the Recipes section of the Member's board. They just compiled some of the favorites and ones that people sent in to be added to the cookbook.

When I first started Feingold, I didn't find that I used a whole lot of the recipes from the recipe board. I found it easier to do a search online myself or search through cookbooks from the library to tailor meals to what my family liked.

I did purchase Jane Hersey's book, "Why Can't My Child Behave?" when I purchased the program. However, it took two weeks to get to me and by then, I already knew why my child couldn't behave. A lot of the information in the book, I had already learned via the message board and the Feingold web site in that two week time (I did a LOT of reading).

However, the book is over 400 pages and very extensive. I just found that when my materials arrived, I had so much to read and go through, that I never had the time to read the book. If you are holding off on purchasing Feingold, this would be a good read though. It covers just about everything. You can read the first chapter of this book for free on Feingold's web site, currently under "Resources."[2]

Appendix

List of Good Resources

People often ask about good books that explain how to do the Feingold Diet. Below are a few. See if you can get them from your library. If your library doesn't have them, ask them to have it sent in from another library (an interlibrary loan). There aren't a ton of books out there specifically on the Feingold Diet. Dr. Feingold wrote a cookbook with his wife back in the 1970's. I haven't read it, but I've heard that it is outdated.

There are a few web sites and blogs by people doing the Feingold Diet. I've listed a few below. There are also several good documentaries that aren't specifically on the Feingold Diet, but on healthy eating in general.

Books About the Feingold Diet

Why Can't My Child Behave? Why Can't She Cope? Why Can't He Learn? By Jane Hersey

The Feingold Cookbook for Hyperactive Children by Ben and Helene Feingold

Why Your Child Is Hyperactive by Dr. Ben F. Feingold

Books on How Food in General Affects our Behavior and Health

The Unhealthy Truth – How Our Food Is Making Us Sick And What We Can Do About It by Robyn O'Brien

What's Eating Your Child? – The Hidden Connection Between Food and Childhood Ailments by Kelly Dorfman

The Crazy Makers – How the Food Industry Is Destroying Our Brains and Harming Our Children by Carol Simontacchi

Books On Saving Money On Groceries

America's Cheapest Family Gets You Right On the Money by Steve and Annette Economides

Cut Your Grocery Bill in Half With America's Cheapest Family by Steve and Annette Economides

I also subscribe to www.moneysavingmom.com (it's free) to receive e-mail notices on sales and coupons for Whole Foods and other stores I shop at.

Books On Time Management

168 Hours: You Have More Time Than You Think by Laura Vanderkam

Eat That Frog!: 21 Great Ways to Stop Procrastinating and Get More Done in Less Time by Brian Tracy

Web Sites

www.feingold.org

Feingold Diet's official web site where you can order the program and get the shopping guide.

www.allnaturalmomof4.com

I'm partial to this one. Also on Facebook -
www.facebook.com/allnaturalmom.

www.feingoldrecipes.blogspot.com

This is my other blog with over 100 Feingold and GFCF recipes.

www.pinterest.com/allnaturalmom4

My Feingold Pinterest boards.

www.reallifeeating.com.

A great blog with a lot of Feingold recipes.

www.100daysofrealfood.com

This is a great site - very informative with some creative ideas on how to eat naturally. They don't do the Feingold Diet but do avoid processed foods, thereby avoiding most artificial ingredients.

www.foodbabe.com

Another great site about eating clean and avoiding heavily processed foods and GMO's. Vani Hari (aka Food Babe) goes beyond Feingold, but there's some interesting information on this web site.

Facebook Group: The Feingold Association of the United States – ADHD Diet

You need to be approved for the group first but they pretty much accept everyone. There are currently over 5,000 members. They are mostly Feingold members but not all. It's a pretty active group and you can post questions and get immediate answers most of the time. They used to not restrict you from talking about brand names.

As of July, 2013, they have changed their policy and now ask that you do not discuss or ask about brand names. They opened up another Facebook group that is for Feingold members only (see below). However, this original group has still remained very active so far and is a good place for those researching Feingold to find out more information.

Facebook Group: Feingold Association of the U.S. – Members Only

The first Facebook group is more active right now but if I have a question about a brand name, I have to post it on the Members Only page. To get access to the Members Only Facebook page, after you become a member, you have to send an e-mail to feingoldfacebook@feingold.org with your request.

There are also a handful of other Feingold Facebook groups. One is for recipes, one is for Feingold homeschooling families, one is called Feingold On a Budget, and there are several more.

Other Web Sites On Health in General

www.mercola.com - This is my favorite. I've been getting his free e-newsletters for a long time. You can go on their web site and search for topics too.

www.naturalnews.com – While the writing tends to be political at times, there are also some really good articles on food, health, and eating naturally. I subscribe to their free e-newsletters.

DVD Documentaries

The following DVD's are about food in the U.S. in general and are not necessarily specific to Feingold. You might want to watch these at a later date when you are not feeling totally overwhelmed by all this new information. However, if you ever need some more motivation to eat healthier, definitely watch these.

Then, just do what you can and take baby steps to a healthier lifestyle. You can find many of these at your library. If they don't have one, they can often have it sent in from another library in your state. A few of these can be found on Netflix, Hulu, or YouTube. New documentaries are coming out all the time.

Super Size Me!

This stars Morgan Spurlock. This movie cracked me up. You might want to watch this first before seeing it with your kids as they do swear and have some off color talk at times. They have a family friendly version if you can find it. It's entertaining and educational. I watched it with my nine-year-old at the time and he liked it.

Sweet Misery

This one is about artificial sweeteners like aspartame and other additives. Very good and does apply to Feingold. Put down your Diet Coke before you watch this one.

Food Matters

This one is about the push to medicate in America instead of looking at diet.

Food, Inc.

Good movie about the U.S. food industry. Makes me want to move to another country.

Fresh – New Thinking About What We're Eating

Often seen as a follow up movie to Food, Inc. Talks about how cattle and chickens are raised and how crops are produced in the U.S. They give examples of changes people can make to eat and live healthier, like growing your own garden.

Forks Over Knives

This one talks about *The China Study* and reversing diabetes and heart disease by eating a whole food, plant-based diet. Great movie. My next goal is to reduce the amount of meat we eat and increase vegetables and other plants.

King Corn

This is about how corn is produced in the U.S. Has a nice piece on how corn syrup is made and what happens when you feed cows corn. We switched to grass fed beef after watching this and we try to buy organic corn products as much as possible.

The Beautiful Truth – The World's Simplest Cure for Cancer

While this talks about cancer, there are some very fundamental principles that apply to everyone who wants to live a healthier lifestyle.

Fat, Sick, and Nearly Dead

Great, inspiring movie. At first I thought this movie was just about losing weight. It's not. Joe Cross goes on a 60-day fruit and vegetable juice fast and is able to eliminate all of his medications and long-time ailments. He also loses weight but the focus of the movie is on how our bodies are meant to be healthy and lean if we feed it the right foods. I had to break out my juicer again after watching this. They are currently filming a sequel to this movie.

Hungry For Change

This is the most recent film out. Loved it! They show interviews with several different people, all of whom have experienced radical transformation in their body size and health, by making a change in their diets. This film does a great job of capturing the whole "food really does affect your health" idea. Most of the other documentaries focus in on one main topic, but this one does a really good job of explaining the big picture.

The point is, whatever you do, continue to educate yourself. Read, read, read! Watch documentaries or YouTube videos. They are continually coming out with new documentaries on food and health. It takes time to really take in all of this information. You do not have to do it all at once. Read a little bit every day about healthier eating and living. What you put into your mind *will* affect the daily decisions you make on what you put into your mouth.

Recipes To Help You Get Started

Below are a few of our favorite stage one recipes to help you get started. I list some brand names. Ingredients and approved products can change at any time, so please be mindful of that and refer to your current Feingold shopping guide to double check any name brands I have listed below. I also sometimes use products that are not officially approved because they will not work with Feingold, but that we use without a problem.

For chicken breasts, look for chicken that has no added broth, is minimally processed, etc. There can be corn syrup in the broth as well if you avoid corn syrup. I like to use organic for health reasons. Many chickens are fed with feed that contain arsenic which ends up in the chicken you buy so I choose to stick with organic chicken. That way I don't have to worry as much about what they may have added to the broth.

We get Organic Smart Chicken brand chicken breasts and rotisserie chickens from Woodman's (here in the Midwest) or sometimes I order organic chicken online from www.blackwing.com.

I order all of our meat from U.S. Wellness right now (www.grasslandbeef.com). We choose to only use grass fed beef. We order their ground beef, roasts, shredded beef, their BBQ sauce, summer sausage, beef sticks (like beef jerky), beef stew meat, steaks, etc. In general, most beef is OK to use. Occasionally, they will have a stamp right on the meat. If yours is stamped, cut off the part of the meat with the stamp.

For a complete list of over 100 Feingold recipes, visit my recipe blog, www.feingoldrecipes.blogspot.com.

Chicken Noodle Casserole

Chicken Nuggets

Chicken Tenders

Garlic Lime Chicken

Hamburger/Steak Seasoning

Garlic Pizza Sauce

Potato Wedges

Vanilla Frosting

French Toast

Pancake Syrup

Smoothies

Pina Colada Smoothies

Gummy Snacks

Lemonade

Oatmeal Raisin Cookies/Ice Cream Sandwiches

Puppy Chow

Chicken Noodle Casserole

8 ounces of cooked noodles   (I use Extra Broad No Yolk Egg noodles)
2 cups cooked chicken, cut into chunks (I use about 3 to 4 chicken breasts)
2 cups chicken broth (I use Pacific Organic Chicken broth)
1 cup milk (I use Horizon Organic)
2 tsp salt (I use sea salt)
1/2 tsp pepper
1/2 tsp garlic powder
1/2 cup butter -1 stick (I use Horizon Organic or Land O'Lakes)
1/3 cup flour (We use King Arthur unbleached but any flour will do)
1/3 cup grated parmesan (Horizon Organic in a bag or buy a block of parmesan cheese and grate in a blender. Store in the freezer.)

Sprinkle some garlic salt over thawed chicken breasts. Cook the chicken breasts. You can either cook in a skillet with about a TB of oil, or place in a 9x13 baking dish in the oven at 375 degrees for about 30 minutes. I pour about a cup or so of chicken broth over them.

Meanwhile, melt 1 stick of butter in a saucepan. Add the flour to make a roux (make it thicker) and stir till smooth. Slowly add the chicken broth (2 cups) and milk (1 cup). Stir till thickened. * Add the salt, pepper and garlic powder.

When chicken has about 25 minutes left to cook, start boiling water for the egg noodles. You'll have to cook them about 8-10 minutes.

When chicken is done, take out and cut into chunks. I drain the broth from the dish and clean it out, then use for the casserole. Be careful. It will be hot.

Combine sauce, chicken and noodles in non-greased 9x13 casserole dish. Sprinkle parmesan on top (optional) and bake in pre-heated 375 degree oven for 10-15 minutes. Sometimes I add cooked peas to this, or you could add carrots too. Kids really like this dish.

Other options: There are lots of things you can do with this recipe. The original recipe called for a can of mushrooms, but I omitted it because we don't like mushrooms. I have added some seasoned bread crumbs (Edward & Sons), or crushed corn flake cereal (Envirokids) mixed with a tablespoon of melted butter to the top when adding the parmesan cheese. I think this is good, but my son freaked out because I changed the recipe and he didn't like the "crunchiness." You could add fresh minced garlic to it or broccoli. Be creative and add whatever your family likes.

Chicken Nuggets

3 cups of rice cereal (I use Erewhon or you could use Barbara's)

2 TB flour (For gluten free, use a GF flour blend without xanthum gum. I use Namaste Perfect Flour Blend.)

1 tsp dried thyme

1 tsp dried sage

1 tsp sugar (I use organic sugar)

½ tsp paprika (omit for stage one)

½ tsp salt (I use sea salt)

½ tsp pepper

½ cup olive oil (I use organic or use Bertolli)

4 boneless chicken breasts

Preheat oven to 400 degrees. Combine the dry ingredients in a food processor or blender. Place a portion of the crumb mixture in a shallow bowl. (I put at least half of the crumb mixture into a zip lock freezer bag and save for later use.) In another bowl, put the oil. Cut chicken into chicken nugget size cubes. Dip chicken in oil, then in crumb mixture.

Place nuggets on a pan lined with unbleached parchment paper (from Whole Foods or online) that has been brushed lightly with oil. Or, I just use a glass baking dish. Bake at 400 degrees for 20 minutes until cooked through. These reheat nicely (400 degrees for about 11 minutes). Let any leftovers cool, then freeze in a zip lock freezer bag.

I double the above recipe and keep the crumb mixture in a mason quart jar to save time when I am making chicken nuggets. These are a staple in our house.

Adapted from a recipe from *Special Eats* by Sueson Vess. Reprinted with permission.

Chicken Tenders

I adapted this recipe from my favorite GFCF cookbook called *Cooking for Isaiah* by Silvana Nardone. You won't need all of the Fritos mixture so I store it in a glass mason jar for when I make these.

10 oz bag of Fritos Scoops (equals about 7 cups)
1 tsp of salt (I use sea salt)
½ tsp pepper
½ cup of olive oil (I use organic or use Bertolli). You can use eggs instead if you want.
4 boneless skinless chicken breasts

Cut up chicken breasts into strips. Pour about half of the Fritos mixture into a bowl. In another bowl pour your olive oil or slightly beaten eggs if you can do eggs. Dip chicken in oil or eggs then coat chicken with Fritos mixture and place on to a slightly oiled baking dish. Cook at 425 degrees for 20 minutes.

Freeze any leftovers. Reheat at 400 degrees for about 11 minutes or until heated through.

Note: Frito Lay recently stopped filling out forms but they were approved for years. We use them without a problem though.

Garlic Lime Chicken

1 tsp of salt (I use Redmond's Real Sea Salt)

½ to 1 tsp pepper (I use ½ for lower oxalates, but recipe calls for 1)

1 tsp garlic powder

½ tsp onion powder

½ tsp thyme

¼ tsp paprika (omit for stage one)

¼ tsp cayenne pepper (omit for stage one)

2 TB butter (Land O'Lakes or organic butter. I use ghee for dairy free.)

2 TB olive oil (I use organic or use Bertolli)

½ cup chicken broth (I use Pacific organic)

4 TB fresh lime juice

Boneless skinless chicken breasts (I use organic)

In a bowl, mix together the seasonings. Sprinkle mixture onto both sides of the chicken breasts. I use about 1/8 tsp of the seasonings on each side of a large organic chicken breast. How much you use depends on how spicy you want it. I like it spicier, but then my kids won't eat it.

In a skillet, heat butter and oil over medium high heat. Sauté chicken until golden brown, about 7 minutes on each side. Turn down the heat and remove chicken and keep warm (put a plate over them). Add the lime juice and chicken broth to the pan and cook for a couple of minutes. Add chicken back to the pan and serve.

I serve with rice and drizzle some of the lime juice mixture over it. I double or triple the above recipe, and keep the seasonings in a jar for when I make this. We make this often.

I adapted this from a recipe on www.flylady.com.

Garlic Pizza Sauce

This is under dinner meals because when you don't feel like cooking dinner, order some pizza! Papa John's Pizza used to be Feingold approved but it went missing from the fast food guide a few years ago. I'm not sure why but many members still get it and have not had any problems. I contacted Papa John's myself and as of 2013, they appear to be clean. You just might want to double check with your local Papa John's to make sure they don't spray their pans with oil that contains BHT or other preservatives.

If you order pizza without sauce, it is stage 1. My son likes to order his with extra cheese, no sauce. Then it's kind of like garlic bread with cheese. I request pizza sauce instead of garlic sauce for dipping because the garlic sauce has artificials, but here is a homemade copycat recipe.

¼ cup of butter

½ TB garlic powder

¼ tsp salt (I use sea salt)

Melt butter. Add garlic powder and salt and stir to combine.

There is another recipe that calls for ½ cup of butter and ¼ tsp of garlic powder. Quite a bit less garlic powder. I guess the moral of the story is, melt some butter, add some garlic powder. If you want more garlic, add some more, and add salt to taste.

Hamburger/Steak Seasoning

2 TB Kosher salt (I use Kosher sea salt)

1 TB pepper

½ TB garlic salt

½ TB onion salt

1 tsp celery salt

Combine all ingredients and store in a small container. I like to use small glass jars. Right before grilling, sprinkle the seasoning over hamburgers or steaks on the top side only. I usually use about 1/8 tsp per hamburger.

I stopped using the grill for health reasons. I now cook everything in a skillet on the stove. I just use about 1 TB of olive oil in a skillet to prevent the meat from sticking.

My son uses Rudi's Wheat Hamburger buns. I can only find these at Whole Foods and occasionally at Trader Joe's. Or we use King's Hawaiian hamburger buns or Whole Foods' bakery's hamburger buns.

My GFCF kids eat hamburgers without buns and dip in ketchup. For pickles, I like Bubbie's bread and butter pickles from Whole Foods (pickles are stage 2). Many regular pickles have yellow dye.

Potato Wedges

My mom makes these for holidays and everyone always asks her for the recipe. She just laughs. It's very simple! I just saw a similar recipe in The Duggars' book, "20 and Counting."

4 organic russet or other white potatoes (about 1 per person)

1/8 to 1/4 cup of olive oil (I use organic or use Bertolli)

1 tsp of salt (We use sea salt)

Pepper (We use the grinder kind that grinds out fresh pepper). I use about 8 twists.

Chili Pepper (optional) I use a few dashes. Omit for stage one.

Cayenne Pepper (optional) I use a few dashes. Omit for stage one.

Wash potatoes thoroughly. You can peel the potato skins if you want, or leave them on. I usually leave them on. They're good either way.Cut the potatoes into eighths lengthwise. Place potatoes in a large bowl and drizzle with olive oil, and mix until all the potatoes are covered in oil. Sprinkle with seasonings and mix to combine.

Place on a dark pan with sides (this is best as the darker pan will help get the potatoes brown and crisp). However, I use a glass 9x13 baking dish. If the potatoes are too overcrowded in the pan, they might come out a little less crisp. Bake at 400 to 425 degrees for 40-45 minutes, or until lightly browned. I flip the potatoes one time about half way through with a spatula.

Vanilla Frosting

3 cups powdered sugar

3 TB butter (Earth's Balance Soy Free or Land O'Lakes or organic butter)

2 to 3 TB rice milk or whole milk (I use Pacific rice milk)

1 tsp vanilla extract (watch for corn syrup and gluten if you avoid those)

Combine all ingredients in a mixer and beat until smooth. Add milk slowly. Add more or use less to get the proper consistency. If it gets too thin, add more powdered sugar.

You can use a zip lock bag to frost. Fill the bag with frosting and cut a small triangle off of one corner. Then squeeze out onto the muffins starting from the outside and working your way around in a circle till you get to the middle. I use a cake frosting tip in the bag to make it look nicer.

We usually add sprinkles. India Tree sells naturally colored sugar crystals (Whole Foods or health food store). I frost banana muffins to use for birthday treats.

To freeze, place frosted muffins on a plate and place in your freezer for about an hour or until the frosting is set, then store in a large zip lock bag. Take one out as you need them. Takes about an hour or so to defrost.

*If you want to color your frosting, use less milk. You can add a pale color using the juice from frozen strawberries or other berry. It will add a very slight flavor as well, depending on how much you use. If you use berries, it would be stage two.

My kids don't care about the color any more, but like to add sprinkles. India Tree makes natural food coloring, but it's very expensive.

French Toast

4 eggs (We use organic cage free but any are fine)

2 TB brown sugar (Domino's Light Brown)

¾ cup milk (We use Pacific Rice Milk or Horizon Organic milk)

1 tsp cinnamon

1 tsp vanilla (I use organic or homemade to avoid corn syrup)

Dash salt (I use Redmond's Real Sea Salt)

Dash of nutmeg (optional)

12 pieces of bread (We use Rudi's Gluten Free or Rudi's Honey Sweet Whole Wheat from Whole Foods. Can also use King's Hawaiian sandwich bread.)

Combine all ingredients in a large bowl or shallow baking dish. Dip and soak bread in mixture. Cook on pancake griddle or pan, greased with butter.

These freeze nicely. Allow to cool and freeze in large gallon size zip lock freezer bags, labelled with the date. I try to lay them individually, not stacked so that they don't get stuck together. Reheat in a toaster or toaster oven.

You could also cut these into strips to make French toast sticks. They also say to use day old bread, so that the bread doesn't fall apart when soaking.

Top with butter or pure maple syrup. We like the syrup from Cracker Barrel. It's half maple syrup and half cane syrup. You can order it from them online or pick it up at one of their restaurants. Or you can make your own syrup. It's not the same as regular syrup but my kids don't complain.

Pancake Syrup

½ cup white sugar (we use C&H or organic but you can use any cane sugar)

½ cup brown sugar (Domino Light Brown)

½ cup water

½ tsp vanilla (watch for corn syrup and gluten)

Put sugar and water into a saucepan. Cover and bring to a boil. When sugar crystals are thoroughly dissolved, add vanilla. Stays fresh in refrigerator for weeks. Warm a portion of the syrup before using. Makes 3-4 servings.

Regular pancake syrup contains artificial flavors and high fructose corn syrup and pure maple syrup is very expensive. I've made this and the kids don't even notice the difference.

We've also used agave syrup. It is a low glycemic and doesn't feed yeast. It has a very sweet taste but some studies say agave is similar to corn syrup so we've stopped using it just in case. I bought a glass syrup dispenser, like those at restaurants, at Bed, Bath, and Beyond. Not necessary, but fun. For pancakes, we like Aunt Jemima Original Pancake Mix (not Complete).

Smoothies

You can do a variety of different smoothies. I get some fresh fruit or Dole canned pineapple and freeze it in zip lock freezer bags. Make sure you label them with the date.

For stage one, I freeze banana chunks, mango chunks, pear chunks (these only last about a month), and canned pineapple. I've also done a melon smoothie with cantaloupe, honeydew and bananas. You could also use kiwi. We do the Pina colada smoothie the most. We also freeze smoothies in popsicle molds to make popsicles.

For stage two smoothies, my favorite is fresh squeezed orange juice (or Simply Orange orange juice) and frozen strawberries. Add sugar to taste if you want. Yum!

My toddler likes berry smoothies with milk, banana, blueberries, and raspberries (stage two). Experiment and see what your kids like best. I don't know any kids who don't like smoothies.

You can also add a nutrient booster like ground flax seed (has lots of Omegas) or other vitamins. We like using the berry flavored Amazing Grass Green Superfood powder (stage two from Whole Foods).

Pina Colada Smoothie

1 to 1 ½ cups of coconut milk (We use So Delicious Original)

2 slices of Dole canned pineapple with about 1/8 cup of juice (frozen works best)

1 banana (in frozen chunks)

½ tsp of ground flax seed/powder (optional)

Add all ingredients into a blender and puree until smooth. If the blender gets stuck, add a little more coconut milk or water until the smoothie reaches the desired consistency. You could also use whole milk or rice milk instead. We've added mango and sometimes cantaloupe to this smoothie before too. One time we ran out of bananas, so I made some mango, pineapple, coconut milk smoothies.

These make great popsicles as they don't stain! We make these often.

Go online to www.amazon.com and look at all the cool popsicle molds. The Annabel Kormel baby ones are my favorite for babies. I recently saw these at Wal-Mart. The Kinderville silicon push-up ones are my older kids' favorite.

Use canned and not fresh pineapple for stage 1.

Gummy Snacks

3 envelopes of Knox unflavored gelatin (by the Jell-O at any store)

1/4 cup of sugar

1/2 cup of fruit juice or pop (open the pop and let the carbonation die down first)

Combine all ingredients in a small saucepan and heat just till sugar dissolves. Pour into molds and refrigerate till firm (about 20 minutes or so). I sometimes grease the molds with coconut oil to make them easier to get out. I use a sharp knife to loosen them out. Store any leftovers in the fridge.

We use 365 Lemon Lime pop, Sierra Mist (not approved but seems OK), or Coke (has corn syrup) for stage 1. For stage 2, you can use 365 root beer, Apple and Eve fruit punch juice boxes, etc. Blue Sky brand has a lot of pop flavors that my kids like too. We get them at Woodman's.

These are really simple but you'll need at least two candy molds from Wal-Mart (craft section usually), or a Hobby Lobby or Michael's. I also bought a gummy making kit from Michael's. It had all the artificial stuff in it, but I threw that out and used the mold because it was of a worm, spider, grasshopper, and frog, and then it also had a nice squeeze bottle to fill the molds with. We got hearts, stars (these are hard to get out), and baby molds (the baby molds had bears) from Wal-Mart.

Lemonade

1 cup sugar (I use organic from Costco or use any cane sugar like C&H)

1 cup hot water

3 to 4 cups cold water (I use 4)

1 cup freshly squeezed lemon juice

Heat 1 cup of water in a saucepan. Add 1 cup of sugar and heat until the sugar dissolves. Add this to a pitcher. Add 1 cup of lemon juice (I usually use about 6 organic lemons). Add 3 to 4 cups of cold water. Stir and enjoy.

You can also add pureed strawberries or raspberries to your lemonade (this would be Feingold stage 2) and throw into popsicle molds.

I have a Pampered Chef pitcher that has the stirrer built in. I make one and a half times the above recipe and it just barely fits in this. But, I usually have kids lined up for some so it works out well. Then I add some ice cubes.

My mom has a lemon tree in her backyard in Florida so she juices lemons in 1 cup increments and freezes them in zip lock freezer bags to make lemonade when we come down. If I have lemons that are about to go bad, I do the same thing.

Oatmeal Cookies/Ice Cream Sandwiches

1 cup (2 sticks) butter, softened (I use Land O'Lakes or Horizon Organic)

1 cup firmly packed light brown sugar (Domino Light Brown Sugar)

1/2 cup granulated sugar (I use organic from Costco or C&H)

2 eggs

1 tsp vanilla (check for corn syrup)

1 ½ cups flour (I like King Arthur flour but any is fine)

1 tsp baking soda

1 tsp cinnamon

½ tsp salt

3 cups Quaker Oats (quick or old-fashioned, uncooked)

1 cup raisins or chocolate chips (optional; omit raisins for stage one. We use Ghirardelli chocolate chips.)

Heat oven to 350 degrees. Beat together butter and sugars till creamy. Add eggs one at a time and beat well. Add vanilla.

Combine flour, baking soda, cinnamon, and salt in a small bowl. Stir, then add to sugar mixture. Mix well. Stir in oats and mix well. Stir in raisins or chocolate chips if using them. Drop by rounded tablespoons onto ungreased cookie sheet. Bake 10-12 minutes or until golden brown. Cool 1 minute on cookie sheet then move to wire rack. Makes about 3 dozen.

My son likes these plain without raisins. We also make ice cream sandwich cookies out of them. Allow to cool completely, then spoon some ice cream in between two cookies. Store in a large zip lock bag. If I know I'm making these, I usually slightly undercook the cookies (about 9 minutes) because they taste better. They don't turn out as good if the cookies are too hard.

Whenever my son takes these to a party, the other kids always want to know where he got the ice cream sandwich cookies.

A few ice creams that are approved are Haagen-Dazs vanilla, 365 brand from Whole Foods, Kirkland Signature from Costco (has corn syrup), and Double Rainbow French Vanilla from Trader Joe's.

Puppy Chow

9 cups of Crispix

1 cup of chocolate chips (Ghirardelli or Enjoy Life for dairy free)

½ cup of creamy peanut butter (JIF, Skippy, or Whole Foods brand)

¼ cup of butter (Land O'Lakes, organic, or Earth's Balance Soy Free)

1 tsp vanilla (check for corn syrup)

1 to 1 ½ cups of powdered sugar

Melt chocolate chips, peanut butter, and butter in a saucepan until smooth. Stir in 1 tsp of vanilla. Pour over 9 cups of cereal and mix well. Cool slightly. If you don't wait long enough, the powdered sugar will dissolve right into the chocolate.

Pour into a large zip lock bag with 1 ½ cups of powdered sugar (or just stir in the bowl). Shake or stir until well coated.

About the Author

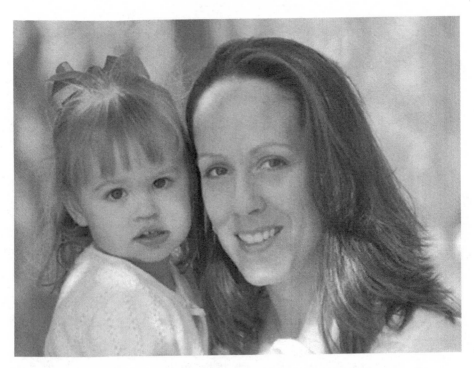

Sheri Davis is a stay at home mom of four kids between the ages of three and thirteen. She and her family reside in Illinois. She has a Bachelor's degree in Business Administration from Elmhurst College. She loves helping families make better choices in food in order to help their loved ones. She blogs about the Feingold Diet, the GFCF diet, autism, supplements, biomed, her faith, and all things natural at www.allnaturalmomof4.com. She posts her favorite recipes at www.feingoldrecipes.blogspot.com.

Find her on Facebook at www.facebook.com/allnaturalmom.

And on Pinterest at www.pinterest.com/allnaturalmom4.

Here's a sneak peek at my next book. There are a few things I wanted to include in this one but couldn't fit it in. I didn't want to overwhelm people with too much information all at once. This next book focuses more on the practical implementation of the Feingold Diet. Title and chapters may change. Look for *How To Implement The Feingold Diet* next year!

How To Implement The Feingold Diet

By Sheri Davis

Table of Contents

Letters to Teachers and Class Parties

A Feingold Birthday Party

How To Deal With Unsupportive Relatives

Ideas for School Lunches

Ideas for Snacks

Ways to Save Time in the Kitchen

All Natural Cold and Flu Care

A Trip to the Doctor

A Trip to the Dentist

Supplements for ADHD

To be notified of future books, visit Sheri Davis' sales page at www.momof4.com.

References

Introduction

1. Wells, S.D. "For Added Freshness" Label Claim Really Means "Added Chemicals" When It Comes to BHA and BHT." 12/16/11. www.naturalnews.com. Natural News. Accessed at http://www.naturalnews.com/034418_added_freshness_BHA_BHT.html

2. "Dyes in Your Food." (n.d.). www.feingold.org. Feingold Association of the United States. Accessed at http://www.feingold.org/Research/dyesinfood.html.

3. Feingold, Ben. "The Role of Diet in Behaviour." *Ecology of Disease*, 1982; 1 (2-3):153-65. Accessed at http://www.feingold.org/bio-medjournals.html.

Chapter 2

1. "Symptoms That May Be Helped By the Feingold Program." (n.d.). www.feingold.org. Feingold Association of the United States. Accessed at http://www.feingold.org/symptoms.php.

2. "Salicylates." (n.d.). Food Intolerance Network. www.fedup.com.au. Accessed at http://fedup.com.au/factsheets/additive-and-natural-chemical-factsheets/salicylates.

3. The GFCF Diet Intervention – The Autism Diet. Accessed at http://www.gfcfdiet.com

4. Cabot, Sandra. *The Liver Cleansing Diet*. Glendale: S.C.B. International, 1997.

5. "Food Dyes: A Rainbow of Risks." 06/01/10. The Center for Science in the Public Interest (CSPI). www.cspinet.org. Accessed at http://cspinet.org/new/pdf/food-dyes-rainbow-of-risks.pdf.

6. "In Europe, Dyed Foods Get Warning Label." (n.d.). The Center for Science in the Public Interest (CSPI). www.cspinet.org.pdf. Accessed at http://www.cspinet.org/new/201007201.html.

7. Hari, Vani. "Food Babe Investigates: How Food Companies Exploit Americans With Ingredients Banned In Other Countries." 2/11/13. Accessed at http://www.100daysofrealfood.com/2013/02/11/food-companies-exploit-americans-with-ingredients-banned-in-other-countries/.

8. Santini, Jean-Louis. "FDA Votes Against More Food Dye Labeling." 4/1/11. Mother Nature Network. www.mnn.com. Accessed at http://www.mnn.com/food/healthy-eating/stories/fda-votes-against-more-food-dye-labeling.

9. "Dyes in Your Food." (n.d.). www.feingold.org. Feingold Association of the United States. Accessed at http://www.feingold.org/Research/dyesinfood.html.

10. "CSPI Says Food Dyes Pose Rainbow of Risks." 06/01/10. The Center for Science in the Public Interest (CSPI). www.cspinet.org.pdf. Accessed at http://www.cspinet.org/new/201006291.html.

11. "FDA Hears From Critics on Artificial Food Dyes. Next Step: Ignore Them." 3/31/11. CBS News. www.cbsnews.com. Accessed at http://www.cbsnews.com/8301-505123_162-44042813/fda-hears-from-critics-on-artificial-food-dyes-next-step-ignore-them/?tag=bnetdomain.

12. "FDA Probes Link Between Food Dyes and Kids Behavior."
3/30/11. www.npr.org. Accessed at
http://www.npr.org/2011/03/30/134962888/fda-probes-link-between-food-dyes-kids-behavior.

13. "Food Additives Could Be Making Your Kids Hyper." 02/08/11.
CBS News. www.cbsnews.com.

14. "Food Counterfeiting: Vanilla Case Study." (n.d.). Virtual Mass
Spectrometry Laboratory. Accessed at
http://svmsl.chem.cmu.edu/vmsl/vanillin/details_1.html.

15. "Japanese Researchers Extract Vanilla From Cow Dung."
03/06/06. www.terradaily.com. Terra Daily. Accessed at
http://www.terradaily.com/reports/Japanese_Researchers_Extra
ct_Vanilla_From_Cow_Dung.html.

16. "Artificial and Natural Flavorings: Avoid Them All!" 05/15/07.
Yahoo Voices. Accessed at http://voices.yahoo.com/artificial-natural-flavorings-avoid-them-all-326680.html?cat=5.

17. Flinn, Angel. "The Gross Truth About Natural Flavors."
11/03/10. Care 2 Make a Difference. www.care2.com. 11/3/10.
Accessed at http://www.care2.com/greenliving/reasons-vegans-read-labels-natural-flavorscastoreum.html.

18. Llaurado, JG. "The Saga of BHT and BHA in Life Extension
Myths." Journal of the American College of Nutrition. 1985:
481-4. Accessed at
http://www.ncbi.nlm.nih.gov/pubmed/4045049.

19. Race, Sharla. "Antioxidants: The Truth About BHA, BHT,
TBHQ and Other Antioxidants Used As Food Additives."
United Kingdom: Tigmor Books, 2009: Accessed at
http://www.foodcanmakeyouill.co.uk/library/content/Antioxida
nts.pdf.

20. Wells, S.D. "For Added Freshness" Label Claim Really Means "Added Chemicals" When It Comes to BHA and BHT." 12/16/11. www.naturalnews.com. Natural News. Accessed at http://www.naturalnews.com/034418_added_freshness_BHA_B HT.html.

21. Eng, Monica and Deardorff, Julie. "Illinois Takes Steps to Ban Trans Fats." 04/13/11. Chicago Tribune. http://articles.chicagotribune.com/2011-04-13/health/ct-met-trans-fat-ban-20110413_1_trans-fats-fats-from-french-fries-illinois-restaurant-association.

22. Botes, Shona. "TBHQ: Why This Preservative Should Be Avoided." 2/14/11. www.naturalnews.com. Natural News. Accessed at http://www.naturalnews.com/031318_TBHQ_food_preservative s.html.

Chapter 3

1. SPD Foundation. Accessed at http://www.spdfoundation.net/about-sensory-processing-disorder.html.

Chapter 5

1. Free Blue Book PDF download. List of Salicylates. Accessed at http://www.fgshop.org/bluepdf.aspx.

2. The Feingold Program (Blue Book). Feingold Association of the United States. Pg 51-52.

3. Hindman, Kimberly, ND. "Tics and Tourette's Syndrome. 06/03/12. www.healingdragon.net. Accessed at http://healingdragon.net/wp/?p=210.

4. "Pica: A Flag For Mineral Imbalances, Especially in The Developmentally Disabled." 02/12/12. Special Needs Kids Go Pharm-Free. http://pharm-freebabiesandkids.com/ Accessed at http://pharm-freebabiesandkids.com/2012/02/12/pica-a-flag-for-mineral-imbalances-especially-for-developmentally-disabled/.

5. "5 Things That Can Help With Tics." (n.d.). New Jersey Center for Tourette Syndrome. www.njcts.org. Accessed at http://www.njcts.org/tsparents/5-things-that-can-help-with-tics.

6. "Gilles de Tourette Syndrome." 04/09/04. Accessed at http://www.newtreatments.org/doc.php/WisdomExperience/177.

7. "Oxalates Control Is A Major New Factor In Autism Therapy." (n.d.). www.greatplainslaboratory.com. Accessed at http://www.greatplainslaboratory.com/home/eng/oxalates.asp.

8. Trying Low Oxalates Yahoo Group. Accessed at http://health.groups.yahoo.com/group/Trying_Low_Oxalates/.

9. Davis, Sheri. "The Low Oxalate Diet." 05/12/09. www.allnaturalmomof4.com. Accessed at http://www.allnaturalmomof4.com/2009/05/low-oxalate-diet.html.

10. "Non-Drug Treatment of ADD/ADHD (Part 3)." 1/14/01. www.mercola.com. Accessed at http://articles.mercola.com/sites/articles/archive/2001/01/14/lendon-smith-3.aspx.

Chapter 6

1. Davis, Sheri. "30 Days of Grocery Shopping, Feingold Style." 04/30/13. www.allnaturalmomof4.com. Accessed at http://www.allnaturalmomof4.com/2013/04/30-days-of-grocery-shopping-feingold.html.
2. Davis, Sheri. "My Feingold Shopping Lists - 2009." 05/03/09. www.allnaturalmomof4.com. Accessed at http://www.allnaturalmomof4.com/2009/05/my-feingold-shopping-lists.html.

Chapter 8

1. Davis, Sheri. "All Natural Couponing." 06/14/11. www.allnaturalmomof4.com. Accessed at http://www.allnaturalmomof4.com/2011/06/all-natural-couponing.html.
2. Economides, Steve & Annette. (2007). *America's Cheapest Family Gets You Right On the Money*. New York: Three Rivers Press.
3. "The Cave Man's Feingold Diet." (n.d.). www.feingold.org. Accessed at http://feingold.org/caveman.html.
4. Davis, Sheri. "3-Day Trial of the Feingold Diet." 07/14/12. Accessed at http://www.allnaturalmomof4.com/2012/07/3-day-trial-of-feingold-diet.html.
5. Vanderkam, Laura. (2010). *168 Hours: You Have More Time Than You Think*. London: Portfolio Trade.

Chapter 9

1. Davis, Sheri. "My Feingold Shopping Lists 2009." 05/03/09. www.allnaturalmomof4.com. Accessed at

http://www.allnaturalmomof4.com/2009/05/my-feingold-shopping-lists.html.

2. Duggar, Michelle and Jim Bob. "The Duggars!: 20 and Counting – Raising One of America's Largest Families – How They Do It." Brentwood: Howard Books, 2008.

Chapter 10

1. Gardner, Amanda. "9 Food Additives That May Affect ADHD." (n.d.). www.health.com. Accessed at http://www.health.com/health/gallery/0,,20439038,00.html.

2. "FDA Urged to Prohibit Carcinogenic Caramel Coloring." www.cspinet.org. 2/16/11. Accessed at https://www.cspinet.org/new/201102161.html.

3. "Food Counterfeiting: Vanilla Case Study." (n.d.).Virtual Mass Spectrometry Laboratory. Accessed at http://svmsl.chem.cmu.edu/vmsl/vanillin/details_1.html

4. "Artificial and Natural Flavorings: Avoid Them All!" 05/15/07. Yahoo Voices. Accessed at http://voices.yahoo.com/artificial-natural-flavorings-avoid-them-all-326680.html?cat=5

5. "Chemical Cuisine." (n.d.). www.cspinet.org. Accessed at https://www.cspinet.org/reports/chemcuisine.htm.

6. "What Is Beta-Carotene? What Are the Benefits of Beta-Carotene?" 11/14/12. www.medicalnewstoday.com.

7. "Add Preservatives to the Packaging Not the Food." 2/17/05. www.foodprocessing.com.au. Accessed at http://www.foodprocessing.com.au/news/10321-Add-preservatives-to-the-packaging-not-the-food.

8. Golden, Beverley. "Can MSG Make You Fat?" 3/24/11. www.sixsimpletruths.com. Accessed at

http://sixsimpletruths.com/2011/03/24/can-msg-make-you-fat/.

9. "Excitotoxins, MSG, and It's Hidden Names." 5/18/11. www. Realfoodwholehealth.com. Accessed at http://www.realfoodwholehealth.com/2011/05/excitotoxins-msg-and-hidden-names/.

10. Erb, John & Erb, Michelle. *MSG: The Slow Poisoning of America*. (2003). Virginia Beach: Paladins Press.

11. Blaylock, Russell, Dr. *Excitotoxins: The Taste That Kills*. (1997). Santa Fe: Health Press.

12. Campbell, T. C., PhD & Campbell, T. M. II. (2005). *The China Study*. Dallas: BenBella Books.

13. Wells, S.D. "Sodium Benzoate Is a Preservative That Promotes Cancer and Kills Healthy Cells." 9/29/11. www.naturalnews.com. Accessed at http://www.naturalnews.com/033726_sodium_benzoate_cancer.html.

14. Woolf, Aaron (Director). *(2007)*. *King Corn, You Are What You Eat*. [Motion Picture]. United States: Mosaic Films Incorporated.

15. "Study Finds High-Fructose Corn Syrup Contains Mercury." 1/28/09. www.washingtonpost.com. Accessed at http://www.washingtonpost.com/wp-dyn/content/article/2009/01/26/AR2009012601831.html.

16. Simontacchi, Carol CCN, MS. "Mineral Deficiencies and Food Cravings." (n.d.). www.diabeteslibrary.com. Accessed at http://www.diabeteslibrary.org/View.aspx?url=Article819.

17. "GMO Facts. Frequently Asked Questions." (n.d.). www.nongmoproject.com. Accessed at http://www.nongmoproject.org/learn-more/.

18. Smith, Jeffrey, M. (Director). (2012). *Genetic Roulette, The Gamble of Our Lives* [Motion Picture]. United States: The Institute for Responsible Technology.

19. Ahmed, Aamena. "The Push to Label Genetically Modified Products." 3/23/14. www.nytimes.com. Accessed at http://www.nytimes.com/2014/03/23/us/the-push-to-label-genetically-modified-products.html?_r=0.

20. "Non-Drug Treatment of ADD/ADHD (Part 3)." 1/14/01. www.mercola.com. Accessed at http://articles.mercola.com/sites/articles/archive/2001/01/14/lendon-smith-3.aspx.

21. "Food Nutrition Labels: Six Catches You Need to Know." 5/11/02. www.sixwise.com. Accessed at http://www.sixwise.com/newsletters/05/11/02/food-nutrition-labels-six-catches-you-need-to-know.htm.

Chapter 12

1. Davis, Sheri. "My Feingold Shopping Lists 2009." 05/03/09. www.allnaturalmomof4.com. Accessed at http://www.allnaturalmomof4.com/2009/05/my-feingold-shopping-lists.html

Chapter 13

1. Campbell, T. C., PhD & Campbell, T. M. II. (2005). *The China Study*. Dallas: BenBella Books.

Chapter 14

1. "Studies On Dyes." (n.d.). www.feingold.org. Feingold Association of the United States. Accessed at http://www.feingold.org/dye-studies.html.
2. Davis, Sheri. "10 Supplements for ADHD." 05/10/12. www.allnaturalmomof4.com. Accessed at http://www.allnaturalmomof4.com/2012/05/10-supplements-for-adhd.html
3. Davis, Sheri. "The Yeast Beast and Our Yeast Protocol." 05/01/13. www.allnaturalmomof4.com. Accessed at http://www.allnaturalmomof4.com/2013/05/the-yeast-beast-and-our-yeast-protocol.html
4. "Leaky Gut/Intestinal Permeability and Enzymes." 08/25/05. www.enzymestuff.com. Accessed at http://www.enzymestuff.com/conditionleakygut.htm.
5. "What Is Dr. Fuhrman's Nutritarian Diet?" (n.d.). www.drfuhrman.com. Accessed at http://www.drfuhrman.com/library/are-you-a-nutritarian.aspx.

Chapter 16

1. Philippians 4:13 "I can do all things through Christ who gives me strength."
2. Colossians 3:23 "Whatever you do, work at it with all your heart, as working for the Lord, not for men."
3. I Corinthians 10:31 "So whether you eat or drink, or whatever you do, do it all for the glory of God."
4. "Maya Angelou Quotes." (n.d.). www.goodreads.com. Accessed at http://www.goodreads.com/author/quotes/3503.Maya_Angelou.

Chapter 17

1. "Love your neighbor as yourself." Mark 12:31b
2. Hersey, Jane. "Why Can't My Child Behave? - Part One." www.feingold.org. Accessed at http://www.feingold.org/Whyone.pdf.

Made in the USA
Lexington, KY
15 September 2016